P9-DWX-896

Springer Series on Social Work

Albert R. Roberts, PhD, Series Editor

Advisory Board: Gloria Bonilla-Santiago, PhD, Barbara Berkman, PhD, Elaine P. Congress, DSW, Sheldon R. Gelman, PhD, Gilbert J. Greene, PhD, Jesse Harris, DSW, C. Aaron McNeece, DSW

Paul Abels, MSW, PhD, is Professor Emeritus at California State University, Long Beach, Department of Social Work. He obtained his MSW from Boston University and his PhD from the University of Chicago. He was Professor and Associate Dean at Case Western Reserve University.

Dr. Abels was a Fulbright Scholar in Turkey and Iran, and he and his wife, Sonia Abels, helped start a school of social work in Lithuania following its independence. He is the author of a number of books and articles, and introduced courses on administration, the future, alternative helping approaches, and narrative therapy for social work.

Dr. Abels has practiced with individuals, families, and groups and did tenant and community organization in Public Housing. He aided his wife in the development of the journal, *Reflections: Narratives of Professional Helping*. His current research is on the use of the United Nations Declaration on Human Rights and how it might be linked to narrative practice, thus providing an internationally appropriate helping approach.

Sonia Leib Abels, MSW, is the Founding Editor of *Reflections: Narratives of Professional Helping*. She is editor of two books in a narrative series: *Spirituality in Social Work Practice* and *Ethics in Social Work Practice*.

Sonia was Associate Professor at the Department of Social Work, Cleveland State University, and Visiting Professor at Haciteppe University, Ankara, Turkey, at Vytatus Magnus University, Kaunas, Lithuania, and at Walla Walla College, Washington, and Clinical Professor at the University of Southern California.

Her research focus is on social connections and social capital. She is currently engaged in building a social work ethics database, sponsored by California State University, Los Angeles, and the National Association of Social Workers, California chapter.

Understanding Narrative Therapy

A Guidebook for the Social Worker

Paul Abels, MSW, PhD
and **Sonia L. Abels,** MSW

 Springer Series on Social Work

YEARY LIBRARY
LAREDO COMM. COLLEGE
LAREDO, TEXAS

Copyright © 2001 by Springer Publishing Company, Inc.

All rights reserved

No part of this publication may be reproduced, stored in a retrieval
system, or transmitted in any form or by any means, electronic,
mechanical, photocopying, recording, or otherwise, without the prior
permission of Springer Publishing Company, Inc.

Springer Publishing Company, Inc.
536 Broadway
New York, NY 10012-3955

Acquisitions Editor: Bill Tucker
Production Editor: Jeanne W. Libby
Cover design by Susan Hauley

01 02 03 04 05 / 5 4 3 2 1

H V
41
.A 254
2001

Library of Congress Cataloging-in-Publication Data

Abels, Paul, 1928–
    Understanding narrative therapy : a guidebook for the social
worker / Paul Abels and Sonia L. Abels.
       p. cm. — (Springer series on social work)
    Includes bibliographical references and index.
    ISBN 0-8261-1382-6
    1. Social service—Psychological aspects. 2. Autobiography—
Therapeutic use. 3. Psychotherapy. I. Abels, Sonia Leib. II. Title.
III. Series.
    HV41 .A254 2001
    615.8'515—dc21

                          00-053828

Printed in the United States of America by Maple-Vail Book
Manufacturing Group

SEP   9 2002

*To Bertha Capen Reynolds, Harry Specht
and all those social workers with courage.*

Contents

data for interpretations, or to be used for making assessments and diagnosis, but not as a tool for change, not as the center of change.

Historically, stories have been used for teaching morality, patriotism, citizenship, and the "American creed." We have had Aesop's fables, the parables, and the lives of heroes and saints, to name a few. We did not recognize their use by the clients as a tool for reconstructing their lives. Oedipus, Electra, Narcissus, and Cinderella became labels that served to diagnose people, and to categorize them, but the stories were not used in the change process. These stories have become part of our culture and shaped our national image as well as our personal lives. Shall we follow the route of Paul Bunyon, who with his great Blue Ox, "Babe," could clear out an entire forest in a day, or should we battle against the machine as signified by John Henry? What do these stories say to us about preserving the ecological balance and the importance of "meaning" in the life of persons?

Psychologists, sociologists, and anthropologists have educated us to know that peoples' views of themselves are sculpted to some extent by their culture as well as by geography, education, and social class. Both complexes of forces are important, or change in the world would not take place. When social work developed the concept of the "dual perspective," it recognized that many minorities experience both their *root* group/family culture as well as the external *branch* culture that may differ from theirs, and that they have to come to terms with both. The power of the mainstream culture is often the most powerful pull. Just as the gang becomes more powerful a pull for the adolescent than his/her family.

It helped us understand the permeability of boundaries, and perhaps their artificiality. We have also learned that some outside shaping forces deliberately subjugate knowledge and persons, for their own self-interest. We know as well, that many approaches to helping people increased dependency, negated clients' strengths, objectified them, and are less effective than we would hope. In addition, we have seen the story of our profession shift away from the social to the psychological and clinical. Our profession realizes that we lack a unifying practice approach that matches our philosophy and professional mission, and that unless we can find a unifying theory and practice, the growing clinical areas of our professional landscape might overwhelm and smother the historical social change aspects of our profession.

In 1993, when Michael White was recognized by the American Association for Marriage and Family Therapy as a master therapist, Stephen

Preface

Just after Christmas in 1648, John Aubrey, out hunting with some friends, rode through the Wiltshire Village of Avebury and there saw a vast prehistoric temple, the greatest of its age in Europe which up to then had remained uncovered. It was not hidden in some remote and desolate spot, for a thriving village stood within its ramparts, nor at that date was it particularly ruinous. Yet Aubrey was the first of his age to notice it . . .

Before Aubrey's visit untold thousands had passed their lives within the walls of the Avebury temple without noticing in its fabric anything more than a random assembly of mounds and boulders. But the moment Aubrey saw it, it became visible to all. Now every year crowds of visitors marvel at the huge scale of the work, the size and precision of the great stones, which three hundred years ago were considered merely an impediment to agriculture and were broken to clear the ground.

Avebury is a stone circle, similar to Stonehenge, and possibly the largest in the world. It is thought to date from the late neolithic period (Michell, 1983, p. 1). When we first read about the discovery of Avebury, we were fascinated by the story, but wondered how something so large and so "obvious" had remained invisible for centuries. Here was something material, solid objects, that can be seen and touched, walked on, through, and past, yet it remains invisible; an artifact that had once served as a major center of thought and belief. What enabled one person to see the gestalt, the totality, the uniqueness of the commonplace, and see it with a new vision? It is a question we can also ask about the evolution of therapeutic thought. What enabled some people to recognize that the power of stories, and narratives, might be used to help people deal with some of their problems? Like Avebury, narrative has always been there, told to therapists by their clients and available to be used if their power could be visualized. We have always walked through and around them. They were always in the background of therapy as well, providing

Madigan wrote:

> White's groundbreaking work of externalizing internalized problem dis-
> course is perhaps his single most important contribution to the field. Since
> then his approach has been heralded by every family therapist organiza-
> tion. He has developed his approach significantly since then and we
> expect it to be a major model in the helping field. (Madigan,1993)

The profession has a great deal at stake in finding the kind of practice
that is effective, but also reflects the profession's values and does not privilege the work with individuals, *nor* the work with larger social units.

In discussing narrative therapy, Bill O'Hanlon in the *Family Networker*,
refers to it as the third wave, the first being the Freudian approaches, the
second cognitive therapy. He suggests that narrative therapy is in the mode
of the postmodern (O'Hanlon, 1994, p.19). Like social work, the psychologists are also searching for a single, successful approach to helping.
Many psychologists are pushing their colleagues to declare the cognitive
approach as its approved methodology. If we were to follow in their theoretical practice footsteps, as we often have, then we too would be reaffirm-
ing the clinical at the cost of the social change schema. Such a step
would be abrogating our historic mission and contract with society.

Narrative practice has arrived on the scene just in time, and the judi-
cial development and use of its precepts offers us a way to replenish the
vitality and joy inherent in a profession that is able to tackle injustice at
many levels.

The message that narrative therapy provides is that the stories that people live by, and that shape their lives, if they are destructive to the person
need to be exposed for the damage they do, and that they can be, and
need to be changed. The vision that narrative provides is that with the
will of the client, and with the help of a worker attuned to the philosophical and practical applications of narrative practice, the person can develop the life story they would like to see for themselves.

Narrative therapy is barely in its infancy, yet has been acclaimed by
leaders in the field as a major contribution. The pioneering and seminal
work of Michael White and David Epson, in their *Narrative Means to
Therapeutic Ends* (1990), provided a base from which narrative could be
explored, amplified, and cultured so that it could be used effectively in a
number of settings and with persons with diverse needs. Narrative therapy
emerged during the postmodern, constructivist movement, helping to
deconstruct privileged helping approaches. It provides the beginnings of

a unifying helping model on which we can build our own, preferred ways of working. It crosses the lines of individual, group, family, institutions, and society. It offers important contributions to the person's understanding of how the problem they face relates to the forces in society, as well as to their own heritage. It helps the person(s) link their lives to the past and to their desired futures. It neither promotes nor emphasizes work with any particular social unit, but uses the supports available to provide the person with room to reauthor their lives. We believe it has the potential to be the quintessential unifying force in our profession.

Narratives have been part of the authors' stories for many years. One of the authors (S.A.), created, and was editor of the journal *Reflections: Narratives of Professional Helping,* for five years. It is currently published by California State University, Long Beach. P.A. has taught narrative therapy at the Department of Social Work at the same university for a number of years.

Our experiences in presenting workshops for field instructors and other practitioners have alerted us to some of the concerns and questions that persons new to the narrative ideas have. Similarly, students in our classes as they interned in their agencies also raised questions as to how to implement some of the ideas they learned. Their feedback, we assume, might reflect some of your concerns as well, as you go through this text. We will present some of the concerns and our comments related to them. We believe that this will be helpful to the reader, who, faced with a new approach, might have similar concerns as they think about using narrative.

You will be the judge of whether or not *narrative practice* is an approach that interests you, and that you care to use. We hope you will proceed with a sense of inquiry, which permits you to examine the narrative ideas carefully, deconstructing them as we propose you do with any model, even those you are familiar with. The research on narrative therapy for the most part is still anecdotal. But what exists reflects an effective approach and one of growing interest. Of course, we hope that as you read on, you will become engaged enough with the approach to think about it carefully, commit, and then use it judiciously.

You may notice that in this last paragraph we use the term narrative practice rather than narrative therapy. We believe that social work is more than therapy and encompasses therapy. Yet in recognition of White and Epston, who named the approach, it is only fitting that it be maintained as the general "label," but to emphasize its expansion, we use the term practice, which in social work is more encompassing.

While our involvement with narrative therapy has been from an academic orientation, we have attempted to present both constructed examples, and practice examples from our students, the literature, and our own limited experience. Efforts have been made to include works of social workers as they have moved into the areas of postmodernism and narrative. We hope that like Aubrey, you will see through the mounds of words, theories, and commentary, to the real contribution to the spirit of helping that narrative practice represents.

Introduction

Where do you come from? Where do you go?
Where do you come from Cotton Eye Joe?
Come for to see you, come for to sing.
Come for to show you my diamond ring.

(Old Folk Song)

Light: The natural agent which emanates from the sun, mental illumination; education enlightenment, knowledge. Pieces of information, facts
which explain a subject; the opinions, information and capacities forming
a person's intellect or mental ability.

FIRST LIGHT

Persons' lives are made up of countless experiences that they organize in
ways that help them make sense of their existence. These events are stories, or narratives that are assigned relative meanings, and make up the
"landscape of the person's life." Jerome Bruner, a leader in helping us
understand the use of the narrative metaphor, notes, "we organize our
experience and our memory of human happening mainly in the form of
a narrative—stories, excuses, myths, reasons for doing and not doing, and
so on" (Bruner, 1991, p. 4).

Persons utilizing a narrative therapist are assisted in revisiting the origins of some of these forgotten, sometime positive, sometimes hurtful, or
unfinished stories, so that they can re-author their lives toward preferred
outcomes. The roots of change lie in the reexamination of the real lived
experiences these narratives provide, the hope for change, and the exploration of desired futures. Shaped in part by culture as well as contextual
life experiences, people think, feel, and behave within the framework of

their continuously developing life narrative. Who you are, what you think, how you learn, how you relate, what you feel, and what you do, are the ingredients forming the landscape of your life narrative. When the incidents in a subplot of the life narrative become too constraining or threatening, truly bothersome, or seriously diminishing of life's meaning, the foundation is set for inquiry which can lead to change. Changes happen in many ways including taking a new job, moving away, joining a group, keeping a journal, becoming depressed, going to the gym, eating more or less, feeling isolated, risking more, going to school, trying something new, and/or taking medication. Some persons seek professional help only when other attempts to change their life do not seem to be working. Helping is a mutual searching out and sharing with people the ideas and resources which help them come closer to the kind of life they want.

The portion of the life narrative a client presents to a social worker frequently leaves out important parts, and a worker needs to be alert to obvious or puzzling omissions, "hearing" them as attentively as she/he hears what is spoken. The untold experiences may contain the seeds which may be valuable in aiding persons to re-author their lives. Unspoken stories may have been forgotten, or appear irrelevant, but may reflect resilience, or a satisfying series of experiences that can serve to reestablish a new direction for the client.

> The woman is about 48 years old, well organized, highly competent, admired, respected by her peers, and attractive. Unhappy with her terminated, long-term abusive marriage, she has begun a new relationship. She asks the worker, "How can I believe this man? He thinks I'm beautiful and charming, and says he will wait for me another year. How can I believe him when my mother was an alcoholic and my father left my mother when I was five years old? My own husband treated me horribly, how can I believe what he (any man) says to me?"

Narrative practice assumes persons' stories about themselves shape their self-views and their behaviors (Bruner, 1990). Some experiences are so entrenched they are featured dominantly in the narrative at stressful life points significantly shaping the person's life. The told story is not the whole story. By looking at the times the woman above thought she did well, then she and the worker will hear about her current executive job and her three children, who have gone to college and attained good positions. Is she the same person now that she was then? Does "self-doubt" keep her from seeing her own accomplishments? In narrative practice, within a context of client-preferred change, the worker assists persons to explore storied experiences so as to discover still unformed, but preferred stories that lie dormant in the subtext of their life narratives, or in normative terms, start the process to "re-author" their lives. Where did she get the idea that she was a failure, because her husband abused her? What part did she play in helping her children do so well? Why does self-doubt want her to distrust others' motivations?

Re-authoring is the process of deconstructing and breaking away from past harmful stories, in this case the uncaring husband, and the feeling of failure and starting to develop a new narrative, constructing a preferred way of life (White, 1991). It minimizes the worker's role as expert and recognizes that no matter how sensitive the worker is, they cannot know what the problem means to the client. It uses unique helping tools such as externalization and mapping of the problem to free the person from feeling that they are saturated with problems over which they have no control. The approach objectifies the problems, rather than the client. Narrative practice supports the client's personal agency in overcoming the problem, searching for elements in the lived stories that amplify unique experiences highlighting times when they successfully dealt with the problems, illustrating their resilience and ability to work on their own behalf. In writing on "human agency," Bandura states,

> The capacity to exercise control over ones own thought processes, motivation, and action is a distinctive human characteristic. Because judgements and actions are partially self determined, people can effect change in themselves and their situations through their own efforts. (Bandura, 1989)

The narrative therapist supports the client's human agency, by minimizing the expert role, and working to discover the submerged knowledge that enables him/her to find openings to write new stories. The discovery of knowledge that was once submerged enables him/her to rewrite the life narrative in a more affirming manner. Most of those exposures to new knowledge come during conversations with clients in which the questions asked examine the experiences that make up the *total landscape* of their lives, not just the current dominant story.

The advantages of this approach according to Michael White, one of the initial pathfinders of narrative therapy, is that it ". . . opens up new possibilities for persons to retrieve their lives and relationships from the problem and its influence" (Tweed Valley Health Service, 1996).

While some of the language in this introduction may seem unfamiliar, clarity shall emerge as narrative therapy is explained further. This first chapter is aimed at grounding narrative in the current scene, and in the historical roots of the helping professions.

Stories are ubiquitous and universal, yet the narrative metaphor, the person's stories as a helping medium, appears new to the profession. Once upon a time, as the story goes when the world was first created, all was dark, and then came light. When we first heard of narrative therapy, we were in the dark. It was a strangely different approach with an unusual language.

We first thought the language pedantic with odd but intriguing ideas. The "strangeness" of the ideas did not fit into our cognitive structure of social work practice, but our dissatisfaction and intellectual doubt about present social work theory and practice pushed us to read more and work harder to understand. We assume it is a universal experience to be uncertain, in the dark so to speak, when faced with strange situations. How to make the strange familiar is an important process. We hope to explain the meaning narrative therapy has to the authors, to transmit that meaning to the reader, to afford the reader an opportunity to gain insight into what's to come, and to illuminate the major themes. Like the overture to an opera faint snatches of melody evolve, and develop more complexity, and are arranged to bring the powerful theme and its variations to completion.

We shall explore a body of practice that started as a therapeutic effort to aid persons by helping them to recognize the contextual nature of their problems. We hope to help you understand why *The Family Networker* proclaimed narrative therapy the "third wave" in counseling, and why the prominent text *Family Therapy* stated that the narrative approach "now dominates the landscape of family therapy," adding that, . . . "it's fitting that the leading approach to family therapy is concerned with the way people construct meaning rather than the way they behave" (Nichols & Schwartz, 1998, p. 397).

Our first two chapters discuss the importance of stories in shaping human behavior, and the narrative metaphor's importance to the therapeutic scene. The idea that persons organize their lives based on the narratives they create from their experiences in the context of their culture is a powerful force in the way they live their lives, a powerful force in the creation of problems they face, as well as a force for change. As persons search for meaning, narratives provide the means to make sense of what is happening to them. The third chapter deals with the profession's history and its relation to narrative ideas. The fourth and fifth chapters examine narrative philosophy, theory, and practice in depth. The remaining chapters cover special areas of social work practice from a narrative perspective.

Every period and every major group in history has had its public story-tellers. Faulkner, Woody Guthrie, Sholom Alcheim, Studs Turkel, El Greco, Leadbelly, First Nation elders, Joyces, the scribes of the Bible, teachers, priests, the writers, the painters, the musicians, and the sayings of the elders. In some places, the traveling folksinger brought the news to the small town, though it was late news, by the time the teller's rounds were completed. It was often the story of some event that the listeners had heard before, but the retelling was important. It was a way to link people with their history and with people from other parts of the country. At a time when there was no writing or people were unable to read, these stories provided values, religious sermons, lessons, and of course communal discussions. The family and tribe made use of this oral tradition to preserve its history. The stories as singing games or plays were also a means of recreation and entertainment. "Tall story" telling was competitive on the frontier.

Traditionally, Sufi teachers believed it was important not to write down their teachings as this made the teachings static creating moral imperatives, too rigid, and inappropriate for different times. They would tell stories that required their listeners to reflect and accept at whatever level of understanding they could. Think about one of my favorites:

> One day a cat teacher was talking to some other cat teachers outside the school. "I don't know what's wrong with those three rabbits in my class," she said. "Yesterday I gave a wonderful lecture on how to catch mice, and none of them paid any attention."
>
> (A Sufi Tale)

Is this a story about teaching, about relationships, about trust, about fear, about adaptation, about cultural understanding, about power, or what? What does it have to do with the helping process? Indres Shah has collected many of these stories and discusses their importance in religion, teaching, philosophy, and as a way of life. (Shah, 1981).

In the study of the Tao, Asian teachers likewise told stories meant for reflection. They created "unanswerable puzzles," called koans, that students reflected on for years. One of the most famous was the koan, "One Hand Clapping." Meditation on these koans was the road to "enlightenment."

In Mario Vargas Llosa's book, *The Storyteller* (1989), an anthropologist works in the rain forests of South America trying to keep the decimated tribes "alive," by retelling them the stories of their creative past. He is both an outsider to the tribes, and an enigma to his "own" people who are limited by the knowledge they can accept.

The songs that Cotton Eye Joe sang were stories of historic importance, of villains, biblical heroes, miraculous events, and nonsense songs. The variety served to insure that everyone in the audience had something to remember about the performance. Joe's livelihood depended on it. Whether or not these "song-stories" were really the "diamond rings" he promised in his song is questionable, but to a community without other means of hearing about the world they may very well have been.

In the beginning was the event! Then came the story. Things needed to be explained and people needed to make sense of things and they still do, and so stories evolved that explained, were retold, and reinterpreted. Every nation, culture, society, organization, family, and individual has a narrative—a series of stories which they have put together, usually in a time sequence that helps them make sense of their lives (Connerton, 1989). It ties them to the past and becomes an integral part of their heritage and their culture. While not usually in the forefront of persons' minds at any one time, these stories weave strands of meaning as part of everyday actions and thoughts. They can come into focus momentarily for a host of different reasons.

If we were to start to explore your story now, right at this point, as you are reading this material, you could reflect on how you came to find yourself sitting wherever you are and reading this book. There is a story here that could be explored. It may be a story of your search for a helping technique that seems to offer something new that you could use which might lead you to reflect on your current practice approach. It may be a story of your teacher requiring you to read this as a text. The story may relate to recommendations from someone you respect, or you might be familiar with the idea from earlier readings. Whatever story you piece together to explain your presence here with this book, it is only part of the story. How did you know that friend? How did you come to be in the class that assigned this reading? How did you come to hear about narrative therapy?

This reading experience that you are now part of is one of a sequence of stories that make up a large part of the total landscape of your life. Some of these events may have only come to mind as you were asked to think about them just now. They are part of the narrative of your life that you may want to be open, or remain hidden. In fact, you may have just come across this book by chance, which also may have a story behind it. For most of you the story of how you came to be reading this book is part of a dominant story of your life, your career, how it evolved, and where you hope it is going. It may be just a hunch, but you are probably reading this to help you become a better practitioner, not a better mother/father or husband/wife. Not to make more friends or for recreation purposes. Those are other stories, some subplots, some dominant, but clearly there are many stories in every life.

Just to carry these reflections one step further, we might ask you to consider the following. How come you are able to read? Can you imagine growing up in a situation where you would not be permitted to learn to read or where you might not have the opportunity to read certain books? Can you imagine a story in which if it was known you could read, you would have your eyes taken out? It did happen during slavery. Your presence at this point is determined in part by the context in which you grew up. How did you come to be in this country? Your ancestors' decisions and stories are an important part of your story, determining, in part, why you are in a position to be reflecting on these ideas now. The way you perceive, accept, or reject some of the ideas you read here has a story connected to it. Your ability to be open to new ideas connects to your life narrative. In the future, if the material you read here turns out to be valuable and useful you may tell others the story of how you came to be a narrative-oriented practitioner.

For this to happen, it is important for the authors presenting a new paradigm to help you examine and to set aside the realistic doubts you might have about investing in a new approach. It is both a puzzle and an adventure to examine a new paradigm. It is exciting to examine new ideas, ones that are helpful. But it is also a puzzle. How good is this, is the author to be trusted, and is it scientific? You may never know to what degree your previous teachings, your familiarity, and comfort with more traditional, accepted models, influence the way you look at narrative. If you are reasonably critical you are right to consider that it may not prove to be better, and may perhaps be even less helpful than the practice you are familiar with, and that you incorporated in your normal day-to-day work. It is therefore important that we present in a clear and particularly concise format the concrete evidence that would make trying out narrative a reasonable decision. This is an important, but often difficult task, because the framework, theory, skills, and philosophy can hardly all be put before the reader simultaneously. More importantly, we believe that not everyone is comfortable with certain approaches, no matter the evidence of their effectiveness. For example, while we are uncomfortable with behavior modification, and would not advocate the use of psychoanalysis by social workers, we would accept their value in certain situations. The introduction of a fairly new approach to helping must overcome previously taught accepted and tested approaches. In addition, the reader/practitioner needs to be able to make sense of narrative practice and this is what we hope to accomplish. The most we can do at this point is to ask you to suspend your judgments, at least for awhile.

Robert Doan, in an article on narrative therapy, presents the following situation: a group of Native Americans and White Europeans are sitting around a campfire, eating, conversing, and telling stories about the creation of the world. "The white men tell their European, Christian, Garden-of-Eden versions. The natives listen politely and comment at the conclusion that they find it very interesting. They all agree it is a good story. They will tell it often to others. They then tell the visitors their creation story. The white men are appalled. Don't they realize there is only one creation story. . . . The white men confer among themselves and quickly conclude that the people they are visiting are non-Christian savages, that it is their duty to save them, to tell them the truth of things" (Doan, 1998, p. 379). The attempts to convince the Native Americans that their story of the creation is untrue led to the killing of many, a story that could be repeated historically in many lands over time. There are many stories about creation. There are many people who believe that persons whose stories are different are not really deserving of respect, and some act on their beliefs in ways harmful to others.

No matter what the group, the story of how the world began was first revealed by a storyteller narrating how it came about. Whether it is the story of creation told in the Bible, by scientific evolutionists, or by a particular culture's narrative of their creation, some explanation of the "beginning" exists in tales, writings, and mythology. There are obviously reasons why each group tries to take into account the unique things that made their existence possible. Anthropologists, philosophers, psychologists, and religious leaders have attempted to explain its importance. Where did we come from? Where are we going?

A SEARCH FOR MEANING

The concept of Narrative emerged to describe the melding of the complex set of meanings from the interaction of beliefs and experiences people use to make sense of the circumstances they deal with as they go through their life transitions. Storytelling is among the earliest methods people used to create meaning in their lives, and is still used today. Linking together events in chronological order helps persons make sense of their own lives, customs, and environment. Holland (1991) notes that,

> . . . the basic process by which people understand the experiences of their own lives and those of others is the narrative. Making sense of experiences requires that each of us formulate a personal story. Efforts to create a meaningful personal story are more than just acts of casual fiction, and the themes that we employ are drawn from the values that undergird our lives. (Holland, 1991, p. 34)

In a discussion related to family narratives, Stern and Szmukler (1999) note that, "Family members are often eager to tell their story, to describe the saga of caring for the ill relative as they struggle to bring into a meaningful form an experience for which there are no clear and definite answers" (p. 354).

Each group's creation stories emphasize the unique reason for their existence, and that uniqueness shapes that group's view of the world. That view becomes such a powerful force, that doubt cast upon the story can lead to dire consequences for any individual or group with a different view. Wars, persecutions, even genocide have been connected to persons' varying stories about "others," their group, and their beliefs. To itemize the many groups who suffered because of their story being different creates a depressing list, calling for efforts beyond time and sanity. The reader only needs to pick up a current newspaper to find his/her own evidence for the truth of our premise.

Similar intense belief surrounds the birth of special individuals important to a particular group. The birth of both Jesus and Moses are two cases in point. Their stories are unique, and in each context, the world of forces around them play an important part in the uniqueness of their birth. The context in which their births occur is crucial to the story. Joseph and Mary must go to Bethlehem because of the tax collection. The baby Moses must be put in a basket on the Nile because of the Pharaoh's mandate to slay Jewish newborn boys. Both are in a particular place because of decisions by powerful oppressors. A sequence of events creates the particular story within the plot. Often the situation is created by the forces which the hero, at some future time, will combat and persevere, as both Jesus and Moses do.

A culture's story of origin greatly influences the actions of its members. It can often determine their life path and influence whether or not they will seek help from a therapist. We know that certain cultures are more likely to seek help outside of the family than other cultural groups, that women are more likely to seek help than men, and that minorities are often less likely to seek therapy than "mainstream" cultural groups. Clearly, cultural stories are important factors that may influence the helping dialogue. Some of these differences are learned culturally, but some are obstacles, real or imagined, that have been determined by social institutions. Institutions and therapists have their own stories and these stories often conflict with the clients' stories. The professional use of "self" is an attempt to take that difference into account. It suggests that workers need to be aware of their own beliefs and how they influence the helping process.

Just as all cultures have a story about their beginnings, people have stories about their beginnings as well. These stories serve to inform persons of their cultural heritage, and suggest and at times narrowly define their responsibilities to the future. These stories of origin suggest something unique about themselves. Whether it is the life of an individual or the life of a group or nation, every culture has a story that in some way explains how they came into being. These stories of how the culture came to be generally reflect positively on their group. While we may now see some of these stories as myths, such as the stories of the Greek and Roman Gods, they were believed to be true at the time and shaped the actions of the people in those societies. When things went wrong, it was because they had offended the gods in some way. Most individual's beginning stories are within the context of the family. As with nations and cultures, the family's stories may often contain myths about its beginnings. At times, families recreate themselves in preferred narratives and claim ancestors who never existed.

The story of Ashley Montague is a case in point. He was a world renowned anthropologist and the author of more than 60 books. He was noted for his United Nations "Statement on Race" in 1949 arguing that "race was a social construct, a product of perceptions about race rather than a biological fact." He was born Israel Ehrenberg on June 28, 1905 in the East End of London, a primarily working-class section. "In previous biographical articles, Mr. Montague apparently said or made it known that he was the son of a stockbroker in the City of London, the financial district, but his father, Charles, was really a tailor, a Polish-born Jew, and his mother Mary, a Russian-born Jew . . . 'I don't know why exactly he changed his name,' Ms. Sperling said. 'He was ambitious to do great things and as Israel, well, that would have been an impediment in British academia' (Ramirez, p. A23). Individuals can be reborn, recreate themselves.

But why would they want to? In Montague's situation, the matter of anti-Semitism appears to have been a critical factor.

Historically, some people attempt to negate the importance of other groups' stories. Postmodernists and constructionists point to the history of particular groups, and the subjugated or ignored material, particularly of minorities, women, and certain ethnic groups. They have urged that the new writings of history have to take into account the biases and omissions of the old stories. Some groups, for example, claim that the Greeks were not the originators of much of their philosophical and democratic thought, maintaining the ideas were borrowed from Egypt (Lefkowitz, 1996). Is the importance of these claims accurate, supported by evidence, or are they politically motivated? Others claim that too much of our history ignores Afrocentric contributions to social thought and that our history texts are too Eurocentric in their orientation. It has been suggested that the DSM was too much influenced historically by German thought. There is no doubt that the phrase, "history is written by the victors," is fairly accurate; as is the statement, "Everything Observed is Observed by an Observer." For example, some might see the Crusaders as liberators, while others perceive them as invaders. Many "facts" are interpretations, influenced by the observer's history, or by political and economic considerations. Admittedly, this may also be true for some of the material presented in this volume. While we try to be objective, we know that we cannot place ourselves out of the context of our own experience. We do try to be humanity-centric. We can also help the reader reflect on some of the things that we talk about. We do this by inserting on a number of occasions a *Reflection*. We hope this serves the reader by raising questions and alternatives, and are links and reminders of some content aspects. For example: *Reflection: If everything is observed by an observer, then isn't it also true that everything written is written by an observer? What is the significance of that idea for the reader, not only for this book, but also for any writing that attests to being nonfiction?*

While the authors write from a postmodern view, we do not suggest there is no truth or that one practice approach is the "true" path to helping. Those with experience in the helping field would be hard pressed to deny the truth of the reality of abused wives, sexually abused children, and crack babies. Those situations exist, they are facts, they are the truth. But even some of these "truths" need to be examined and deconstructed. Some who claim to have been sexually abused as children were not. What are the dangers in labeling an infant a crack baby? We believe that some things taken as the truth be examined. Who puts them forth as truth? Who were the authors? What did they have to gain? What was the context at the time the material was presented? Were there biases related to gender, ethnicity, age, or culture that might have framed the material in a way that ignored other facts? Who suffers from these "truths?" Why was a particular idea privileged over others? Why now?

We suggest that the knowledge that shapes our own practice directions needs to be examined carefully. All social science models are subject to error, and none should just be accepted and given a privileged place at face value, which is particularly true in situations where persons' lives and welfare are at stake. Furthermore, we believe that some practice approaches are more appropriate for use in our profession than others—approaches in which the worker is not the authority as to what is best for the client, or where the client is seen as the problem or labeled codependent.

Although we believe narrative practice is evolving into a powerful, respectful, and appropriate vehicle for social work, we do not suggest it replace approaches that work well for the client and the worker. The developing research that supports many of narrative therapy's ideas, is still thin, and until it stands the test of rigorous experiential scrutiny it must be used carefully. The narrative work with clients, as all practice, needs to be documented with care. We also believe that there is not one practice model that will serve the worker in all situations; and that it is important to be familiar with a range of helping approaches, even those which might not seem to fit a set model. In fact, like Lynn Hoffman (1998), we would agree that we might be better off to avoid "a model." In keeping with that view, we suggest that although we are putting forth Narrative as our preferred approach to helping, it needs to be examined just as carefully as other models need to be evaluated. The same questions need to be asked that are asked of other approaches. Who are its proponents? Who gains, who loses? What is good about it and what not so good? Who might most likely be helped by the narrative approach? Who might not? Can it unify the profession or does it serve a particular subsystem more ably than another, a particular type of client, individual, or group? What are the consequences for the client as far as respect, freedom, and accomplishment of desired ends? The reader may find some of the answers within this text, or better yet, within their own reflections and practice. They may also want to modify the approach as they experience it, adding certain practices that they feel would enhance the helping. At the same time they may avoid certain techniques that they are not comfortable with, or that seem not to work with the particular clients they serve. The idea of social work to individualize the client is still a basic practice principle.

A word about the term "therapy," and our preferred use of the term practice. Language is a powerful tool. Our profession has always worried about the proper use of terms, seeking those that would not be seen as harmful to the client, either by others, and/or by the client him/her self. Labels create stereotypes and categories in ways that are often countertherapeutic. We are very sensitive to the harm that labels might lead to, particularly for the persons labeled with terms that create "stigma" (Goffman, 1963). Stigma is an attribute that is discrediting of the person. Those stigmatized are often seen as less of a person than others are, usually those doing the labeling. Stigma can act as a form of social control. By labeling a person mentally ill, or a convict, or an alien, they are put in jeopardy. Goffman notes that some persons who suffer lengthy periods of being stigmatized start to take on that attribute in all social situations and exhibit behaviors that support the outsiders' views. Frequently, when persons experience stigma, they accept that assignment and experience shame and self-loathing.

Preventing client stigma was a major concern decades before the concept of a "politically correct" language was even a thought. Seeking help is still stigmatized by some and therapy carries connotations of treatment and mental illness. It is closely aligned with the medical perspective and with being "sick." This is certainly not the case for most of the persons who social workers deal with, where family problems, self-esteem, searching for education, and economic security are causes for seeking help.

Jessy Taft, back in 1932 in her classic contribution to our profession, *Social Work Theory*, wrote,

> The word "therapy" is used instead of "treatment" because in its derivation and in my own feeling about the word, there is not so much of manipulation of one person by another. To treat, according to the dictionary, is to apply a process to someone or something. The word therapy has no verb in English for which I am grateful; it cannot do anything to anybody, hence can better represent a process going on, observed perhaps, understood perhaps, assisted perhaps, but not applied. The Greek noun from which therapy is derived means "a servant," the verb means "to wait." I wish to use the English word "therapy" with the full force of its derivation, to cover a process which we recognize as somehow and somewhat curative and if which, if we are honest enough and brave enough, we must admit to be beyond our control.

Without going into the derivation of words as Taft did, we intend to use the term *practice* rather than therapy as we discuss narrative even though the term therapy is not used in a narrow clinical manner by the narrativists. Our reason is that therapy has come to be identified with "clinical" practice solely and increasingly with private practice and not public social services or with social action both of which make up the matrix, odd as it may be, of social work. We believe that narrative most assuredly encompasses clinical practice but that its strength as a helping approach is that it offers a broad range of change opportunities, including community organization and institutional social change. It can have an important impact on society and culture as it utilizes processes that go beyond the "treatment" in an office setting and into the real life of the persons served. At its core, it is the *practice of liberation,* aiming towards individual and societal fulfillment and social justice. In our exposition on narrative we will try to present both the positive aspects and the limitations of the approach as we, and other authors have seen them. All the authors have common ground on the idea that life is narrative. We also know that even when all other things are gone, we still have our story, providing we have someone to tell it to. It is important to know that in social work, as in other professions, the story does not always have a happy ending. There will be times when regardless of what the client and social worker are able to do together the external forces may be so destructive as to negate any of the positives that could take place in the client-worker matrix. It will be important then, to work on those external forces, and as Allen Wheelis, a postmodern psychiatrist, suggested, when things aren't going well with a client, we need to try harder, and try something different. We are reminded of a song we used to sing at camp:

> This little light of mine. I'm going to let it shine.
> This little light of mine, I'm going to let it shine.
> Let it shine, let it shine, let it shine.
> Don't you let them blow it out, this little light of mine.
>
> (Folk Song)

The light that needs to be maintained is our humanness, individuality, resilience, and courage; the lights are determined by the stories we have incorporated into our beings. Where have we been? Where are we going? These are the same questions asked of Cotton Eye Joe. They are the questions you can reasonably ask of us. We hope we can provide the answers as we go along. We may not be able to show you our diamond rings, but we can sing you the story of narrative, with some of its variations, and hope it remains harmonious. We also need to caution you that it is an unfinished symphony.

2

Making Sense of Our Lives

"Stories are important. They keep us alive, in the ships, in the camps, in the quarters, in the field, prisons, on the road, on the run, underground, under siege, in the throes, on the verge—the story teller snatches us back from the edge to hear the next chapter. In which we are the subjects. We, the hero of the tales. Our lives preserved. How it was: how it be. Passing it along in the relay. This is the work I do: to produce stories that save our lives."

(Toni Cade Bambara)

Story: A true narrative, or one presumed to be true, relating to important events and famous people of the past; a historical account or anecdote . . . a person's account of his or her experiences or the events of his or her life.

THE DYNAMICS OF STORIES

Imagine that you are in the South African courtroom of the Truth and Reconciliation Commission. The country has just emerged from apartheid, the most destructive period in its history. Sitting in the courtroom are white and black South Africans. The oppressors, mostly white, and the oppressed and victimized, mostly black. Both groups tell their stories of the atrocities committed primarily on black South Africans. The Commission's members hearing the testimony are the leaders of the new South Africa, including Archbishop Tutu who won the Nobel Peace Prize in 1984.

The local and international press extensively covered the first public hearings held by the commission in 1986. Ms. Antjie Krog, a white South African reporter, covered those hearings. These brief excerpts from her book *Country of My Skull* (1998) give us some clues as to the importance of telling one's story, and can help us reflect on how social injustice leads to personal problems.

The following testimony, presented to the tribunal, is from a black South African. The hearing room is packed, but there is a hushed silence as people stretch to hear the words.

> This was the last thing I saw; Barnard standing next to his car. He spoke Xhosa like a Xhosa. He pointed his firearm at me. I felt something hitting my cheek. I felt my eyes itching. I was scratching my eyes and yelling for help. Since then I've been blind and unemployed and alone and homeless. But today, today it feels as if I can nearly see. (p. 29)

> Ms. Gobodo Madikizela (panel member): How do you feel Baba, about coming here to tell us your story?
> Mr. Sikwepere: I feel what—what has brought my sight back, my eyesight back is to come back here to tell the story. But I feel what has been making me sick all the time is the fact that I couldn't tell my story. But now I—it feels like I got my sight back by coming here and telling you the story." (p. 31)

The transformative power of telling their stories, part of the narrative of their lives, frees people to imagine their new stories and move on to productive lives. A deep, optimistic hope lies in the healing potential of the public confession of those complicit in committing atrocities and the public documenting of the stories of those so deeply harmed.

The oppressors told the stories of their role in the brutality of apartheid, and sought forgiveness. Doing so meant that they could move on to new, preferred life stories, partially cleansed from the evil they had committed. The process of telling and knowing that their stories were being heard by the world meant that they were important, vital, and autonomous persons with an important contribution to make to the future of their country. The oppressed made public the brutality they had experienced. They could see themselves as human beings and became more able to gain a sense of what had happened to them. They had been assigned the role of tortured actors in the subplots of the national plot to keep them subjugated. This was revealed time and time again, testimony by testimony by those who had conceived of apartheid. The oppressed separated themselves from the oppressors through the horror of their stories, and the nobility of their survival. Face to face with those who had controlled their destiny, now on equal footing, person to person, they reaffirmed themselves as persons. They had survived the efforts to dehumanize and subjugate them. It was a rebirth for them and the nation. Making the stories public was a vital and necessary process that permitted South Africa to heal.

It is the amazing power of stories to aid in the helping process, when used in narrative practice, that led *The Family Networker* to highlight it as the "third wave" in therapy (O'Hanlon, 1994). And as we have noted, it has motivated the authors of a leading text on family therapy to state that it currently "dominates the landscape of family therapy" (Nichols & Schwartz, 1998, p. 397). One of those authors has also commented further on the positive potential of narrative therapy (Schwartz, 1999). As you read on, you have the opportunity to make your own judgment about the accuracy of these views.

As advocates for an approach that seems to us more likely to reflect our professional experiences with clients, we are impressed by some of the basic philosophy on which narrative theory is founded. Aside from its compelling originality, there are five major reasons for its increasing popularity. First, it is our view that the narrative approach significantly reflects the historic mission and purpose of the social work profession. Second, we believe that narrative practice offers unique practice principles and a socially contextual perspective, which gives life and rationality to the practice it offers. That is, one can see that the practice principles follow directly from the theory and the philosophy. Third, and perhaps most crucial, it deals with the person's situation in its social context. Fourth is its synergistic use of client(s) and worker in mutual aid, rather than presenting the worker as the expert. Finally, it minimizes client self-blame and offers ways for persons to use their energies instead to move in their desired directions.

The profession's several practice approaches have had a good deal of staying power over the years. The selection is varied—there have been functional, Freudian, solution-oriented, behavioral, psychodynamic, cognitive, interactional, existential, and various other family therapy "models" which had some major influence, particularly the structural and strategic therapies. Some approaches have had a tenuous, often fleeting existence, such as inner child, co-dependency, eye-movement therapy, and tough love. Some have been found unhelpful and others abusive of clients, or dangerous. We suggest that the variety of approaches does not reflect the profession's creativity, but rather the need for a more centered and universally effective practice, a practice in which client and helper are united in the helping effort, human and human (Friedman, 1993).

When persons understand that the stories they tell in conversations with the helper are not reflections of them as incompetent, or a less whole person, it increases their capability to talk more freely. They do not feel judged. When they recognize that often the problems they face emerged from social forces, society created circumstances that enforce negative views of themselves and make them objects for study, or pity, they gain new confidence. These life stories and how they influence the change process are at the heart of the narrative approach. They aid persons to find meaning in their lives and to make sense of the complex events leading to their present situation. It facilitates re-authoring and provides an opportunity to shape the story of the desired future.

Narrative practice deals with stories that shape the lives of persons and helps them examine how these stories might both help and hinder them from achieving what they seek (Parry & Doan, 1994; White & Epston, 1990). Often a specific aspect of their current story has brought them for help; it is the first story the helper hears, and the one to which he/she must respond. For the moment, it is the most important event in the person's life, the reason for their concern, and the reason why they want help. Examining with the client where these stories came from assists in exploration of the social context that puts the story in some sequence, and gives both worker and client knowledge of the lived life of the person.

Since most therapies start with the client telling the story of why they have come for help, the reader might be wondering, "so what is new about what the narrative practitioner does? What do they do that is different? How do they use the stories? What is unique about their perspective?" For a start we might respond that the stories are examined with the client in a manner that helps to identify the sources of the story, how it came to be so disconcerting to the person. While this helps the worker get a sense of direction, it also can help the client understand the social forces that shape the stories, and influence and shape his/her views of the world and subsequent actions which might be taken.

It is important to point out that these are the clients' stories, not stories that the worker tells the client to make them feel better, or to make a point. The worker explores with the clients how their lives are shaped by the stories they believe about themselves, accurate or not. A basic part of narrative practice is to help the person understand that these stories frequently come from powerful forces, and/or from others with something to gain by creating influencing narratives, true or not, that help them maintain power or subjugate others. The reasoned policies undergirding the imposition of apartheid were meant to insure the total subjugation of the black South African population. Less extreme examples can be seen in our own educational system, particularly in communities where some students are channeled into industrial trades-oriented tracks, and others into college-oriented tracks. The difference is often related to class or ethnicity. Education went beyond increasing knowledge but is often a form of social control. Being late to school incurred relative punishments. Being tardy became a "dirty" word, as one goal of being on time had to do with educating future workers for good work habits. We were all taught to draw inside the lines.

SENSE MAKING: THE POWER OF THE NARRATIVE

The power of stories to influence people to shape the formation of a nation, and to demonstrate the importance of justice, was branded into the world's consciousness by two of the most significant events of the twentieth century, the Holocaust and Apartheid. The stories of the Holocaust and Apartheid serve to remind of us of the dangers of genocide and ignoring national brutality. The international reactions to such outrages have intensified and quickened our response to such dangers and our press for social justice, as evidenced by the boycotts and the evolution of a "new" South Africa. In the fall of 1993, Apartheid officially ended in South Africa and the nation faced the task of forming one country out of a cesspool of hatred, atrocities, severe economic inequality, and subjugation of black South Africans by the white minority. Through its strategy for reconciliation, the extraordinary process of the public telling of personal stories and testimonies of the subjugators and those subjugated, the torturers and the tortured, and the killers, and the families of the killed came forth to testify. It was an effort in public healing. It was an effort to save the country and help persons make healing connections with each other.

Some of the oppressors came to ask for forgiveness, some to maintain their status and perhaps their way of life. Many of the oppressed came to express themselves, and to establish that even if they could not make sense of what they had been put through, they were human. Their expressions exemplified a search for meaning and the search for self. All testifiers told what happened and what they did to others or what was done to them. Some sought forgiveness, others sought retribution. It was not retribution in the sense of demanding punishment, but the internal retribution that comes from freeing oneself from the bondage and floggings of inhumanity. The telling made them authors of their own lives, an agency for themselves. How did this remarkable re-authoring of a country toward a new future take place? Why this method?

As the end of Apartheid in South Africa drew near, there were a series of negotiations to form a new government in South Africa. Both groups, the traditional Apartheid leadership and the Mandela coalition government, agreed there needed to be a healing process which might, among other things, provide amnesty for those who had committed political crimes. One of the major requirements was that those seeking amnesty would need to talk about what they had done, to testify, and seek forgiveness. It led to the creation of The Truth and Reconciliation Commission.

People of all political persuasions who were interested in a peaceful transition for the new South Africa believed that if there were to be trials and punishments the process of peaceful unification would be doomed. There would be an intractable power group of the white power structure, resisting any efforts at change, because it might mean they might end in prison or worse. Thus, there was an agreement that those admitting their acts, and claiming they did it for political reasons, and asking for forgiveness, could be absolved.

While this in itself was an unusual political process, it went even further. A significant part of the hearings provided for open testimony from all those who wished to speak, including those who had been harmed. They would be permitted to tell their stories if they wished.

There was recognition of the healing power of the narrative. It was more then catharsis, but a belief that the person, the country, could not survive unless the stories could be told. While Archbishop Tutu was a strong believer that forgiveness was important, he also promulgated the belief that through persons telling their stories there would be a release of pent-up emotion and bewilderment. The telling could lead to the freedom to rebuild the nation. These stories were of oppression, murder, torture, slander, and bewilderment. Many of the victims could not, even today, understand how people could treat them the way they had. The many hurts of being called vile names, treated as subhuman, denigrated, seeing family and friends murdered, and being powerless to do anything about it led them to believe that they were worthless, not to be taken into account. As we examine the reconciliation procedures a little further we see how this process worked.

Mr. Sikwepere is seated before The Truth and Reconciliation Commission of which Archbishop Tutu is the chair. Mr. Sikwepere is making a statement about a police raid in which he was questioned by Bernard, the officer (nicknamed the Rambo of the Peninsula), about why he was not permitted to stand around speaking to some of his friends.

"The white man said this in Afrikaans—'you are going to get eventually what you are looking for. And I am going to shoot you' . . . After that I heard a loud noise, it sounded like a stone hitting a sink. But I decided not to run. I decided to walk. Because I knew that if you ran you were going to be shot. When I arrived at the place where I thought now I am safe, I felt something striking my cheek. I couldn't go any further. I felt somebody stepping on my right shoulder. And saying, 'I thought this dog had died already.'"

Ms. Gobodo-madikizela: "Baba, do you have any bullets in you as we speak?"

Mr. Sikwepere: "Yes, there are several of them. Some here in my neck. Now my face feels quite rough. It feels like rough salt. I usually have terrible headaches."

Part of the belief behind the commission's establishment was that being able to create a new South Africa depended on the ability for all those who suffered to be able to tell their stories. This has a strong verisimilitude with narrative therapy that helps people re-author the stories of their lives toward preferred stories. The black South Africans were called "dogs" because this was a part of the denigration and the subjugation. The objective was to make them feel less than human. That was the story those in power wanted them to accept about themselves. That was the context that created the problems.

Narrative therapy's roots, its philosophy, goes back to an understanding of how people's stories of their lives—the things they have come to believe, been taught to believe, or been forced to believe—shape their lives (Bateson, 1972; Foucault, 1965, 1980; Reynolds, 1934). Are we too redundant in making this point? We think not, because this is at the heart of the approach. The opportunity for people to tell these stories, and to recognize both the truth and the falsehoods behind these stories has become one of the basic tenants of narrative therapy. In discussing Elie Wiesel's memoirs, John Carrol (2000) points out the importance stories play in Wiesel's life.

He was 16 when American soldiers found him among the living dead of Buchenwald. In his new book he writes of the understanding he and his fellow inmates had come to: "The one among us who would survive would testify for all of us. He would speak and demand justice on our behalf; as our spokesman he would make certain that our memory would penetrate that of humanity. He would do nothing else. (Carrol, p. 10)

There are people who would prefer not to have such stories disseminated and would like to subjugate this knowledge. Some claim the Holocaust

never happened, or the numbers were exaggerated. What is the importance of negating the "truth" of the Holocaust? Or the self-serving roots
of Apartheid? Why do some powerful people want denigrating stories to
be disseminated? Making subjugated stories public helps the victims
understand what has been done to them. It can also help persons understand how myths, stories, and lies can be used in strategic ways.

Throughout the history of social welfare there have always been negative stories. Blaming parents, singling out "welfare mothers," or labeling
them cheats after a handout, immoral, lazy, and so forth. These stories
when repeated often enough are not only accepted by the population at
large, but often by the subject of the stories themselves.

In most cultures, and certainly in all times, there have been sustained
beliefs that certain groups of persons are more valued then others. Stories
are told about those "lesser" groups that are intended to promulgate their
"inferior nature." In our time, in our country, these groups have included
ethnic minorities, religious groups, women, gays and lesbians, and those
with some form of disability. To some degree the poor as a group are also
considered deviants since they do not possess what others have (Illich,
1973; Kozol, 1995).

As we examine narrative therapy we will see that much of its philosophy
relates to the social use of power and control. The postmodern movement,
and particularly the work of Foucault (1980) focuses on the history of institutional power structures, how power controls language, and how language
influences views of persons and their views of themselves and others.

The postmodernists challenge the things we have come to believe
about the world and about ourselves. In a sense this is the nature of
reflective practice with which social workers have become familiar through
the work of David A. Schon (1983), *The Reflective Practitioner.* Note the
themes in this article on postmodernism:

> A society enters the postmodern age when it loses faith in absolute truth—
> even the attempt to discover absolute truth. The great systems of thought
> such as religions, ideology, and philosophies have come to be regarded as
> "social constructions of reality." These systems may be useful, even respect-
> ed as profoundly true, but true in a new, provisional, postmodern way. Few
> expect that one truth ought to work for everybody. (O'Hara, 1995, p. 22)

The nature of the helping process in our field is unique in that it
depends for the most part on the communication between the person
and the helper. There are no material tools, no "medicines," just an

examination with the helper of certain things that may be influencing their lives, and looking for ways to help them either modify or obtain resources that will influence the direction of their lives toward preferred futures. Increasing the knowledge of both worker and the client are the mechanisms driving the change process. It is a work of mutual exchange of knowledge and understanding. With this increased knowledge and understanding the story is thickened and the plot redirected.

THE UBIQUITOUS NATURE OF STORIES

Narratives have moved from the domain of literature into the helping professions and are now moving to the sphere of big business and the corporations. Some companies have made use of stories in a number of ways. Many corporations have published books, telling the story of their organization; often these are romanticized and mythical. One use of an organization's founding story is as an historic symbol to influence the workers and the consumers of the product of its importance, or its contributions to the growth of the country. The Ford motor company, for example, uses the story of Henry Ford's development of the first assembly line, and the history of the "Model T," as an important part of Ford's image creation. Of course, it attempts to ignore negatives such as the hiring of goons to break strikes, the dismal failure of the Edsel car, and not reporting tire blowout records.

Industry uses stories in other ways as well, such as an article in the *New York Times*, headlined "It was a Dark and Stormy Sales Pitch, and Maybe It Worked—Companies Learn the Value of Story Telling" (Quinones, 1999). The author discusses how stories are being used to help companies and their sales people make more sales. The head of the company that trains these business people notes, "But it can be difficult to persuade a roomful of strangers that stories about personal experiences can help them achieve business goals." In discussing why he relates some anecdotes about his business, one respondent said, "They're interested in the journey and what it took to get there."

THE STORIES OF LIFE

Batman looked at the large plastic globe that separated him from Superman. He fingered it lightly at first, then began to smash at it with his fist. He then started to kick it and it began to crack.

"He's breaking your globe," the Green Hornet yelled at Superman, who turned just in time to see his globe crack into three large pieces. "I'll kill you, kill you," Superman screamed at Batman. "I'll kill you, kill you. . . . I'm going to tell your father on you."

The worker-driver pulled the station wagon into the nearest parking lot, stopped and turned to the boy. (Abels, 1973, p. 37)

This adventure was the first time I really understood how important stories are in the lives of people. I was working with a group of 10- and 11-year-old children who were labeled mentally retarded. This was in the less enlightened years of the late 1960s, when labeling people was unquestioned and the impact of the labels on the person was not a significant concern, nor even considered.

Each of the six children in the group assumed the name of a comic book hero of the time. Interestingly enough some of those characters still exist, stimulating the creativity of other children. Our group had Superman, the Green Hornet, Batman, and assorted lesser-known heroes. During the two or three hours that the group met each week, they often assumed these characters' persona, not that they tried to fly or leap across tall buildings, but they acted differently. They would become more assertive in their interactions with each other and with the worker. They were very different than at our earlier meetings, when they were their "real selves." They were even themselves during the first five to ten minutes prior to the start of meetings while we waited for all members to arrive. They became more assertive when the meeting began. Assuming the roles of these characters seemed to give them a sense of power and control over their lives.

At the time, I recognized the importance these role assumptions played in their lives, and there was no attempt on my part to say, "be yourself." The fantasy was accepted and at times the group discourse included members addressing themselves by their heroic names. At times even the environmental context changed. The car which took us to various sites would become a batmobile or a space ship. The visit to the ancient armor room at the museum stimulated further heroic fantasies of fighting "bad" knights. Of course I had no awareness at the time of things like narrative therapy, or how to make use of the stories in a helping way. My awareness stopped at the recognition of how important being those characters were to these children. While I recognized that it gave them a sense of power, we only briefly discussed why they wanted to be Superman, or Batman. Nor did I give much thought to why a particular child chose a particular character. What did they see in that person? Neither did it occur to me to consider that the African-American child chose a white hero. When I think back on it, I did not know of African-American comic book heroes in those days. In fact, until recently none have appeared in the weekly comics either. Perhaps, I had not paid enough attention to my course work in graduate school, but things such as racism and the meaning of stories did not seem to be part of the curriculum. I made use of the stories to help at the most obvious level. It gave the children something to do, and helped them make connections with each other. It provided friendships that they didn't have at school or home.

I am reminded, however, of an earlier time, when stories had been an important part of the lives of children I worked with. I had been the program director at a camp for handicapped children years before. They particularly liked me telling them the Brer Rabbit stories. They were excited about how Brer Rabbit would outsmart the Fox. At that time I had some glimpse of the idea that stories in which the theme showed the "underdog" outsmarting the powerful might have special meaning to these children. But these never became part of a dialogue to explore their feelings. I make a point of discussing my lack of awareness, because I believe it is relative to our concern about reflecting on our practice. We have a lot of knowledge which we do not use, because we often do not reflect on what the meaning of the experience might be to the client, as it is being lived.

For these children at camp, and for the boys in my group, the stories of their lives did not include many affirming social experiences. The two weeks camping was an exception. For the boys, having a club of their own meeting each week was another exception. If I were working with these former group members now that they are adults, we could look at these early "good" experiences as a way to help them look at their abilities to be creative and to interact well with others. This could be a factor in helping them understand their own powers to reshape the future, or in White's terms to help them "re-author" their lives. This might lead to their desire to participate in groups in which they could help set the direction of the group, take leadership positions, and/or have other persons with whom to make connections and relate. This looking at other stories in the person's life, in which they were able to handle certain situations, is a tool the worker uses to help the client recognize his/her own powers.

An interesting use of stories to demonstrate how a narrative can be used to overcome conflict and rivalry among two groups of youth is described in Muzafer Sherif's article, *Intergroup Conflict and Cooperation: The Robbers Cave Experiment* (Sherif, 1969). The setting is a summer camp. Two groups of boys are placed in situations of competition with each other and are urged into conflict by their counselors. During campfire get-togethers, the campers have been told of a buried treasure in a cave a few miles away, buried from an old robbery. The story is expanded and made more exciting by the promise that the groups can take an overnight trip to try to find the treasure. On route they are placed in a situation where the bus breaks down and the two groups are forced to cooperate with each other in order to get to the cave. The conflicts between the groups are forgotten as they work out the problem of getting to their goal together.

THE CALL OF STORIES:
THE STORIES WE LIVE WITH

Robert Coles, a psychiatrist and Harvard professor, has written extensively on children's lives, the importance of stories, and how stories shape the lives of the therapist, the client, the student, and the teacher. His focus on the moral issue of living requires students to do community service and read novels, short stories, and poems. He notes that through these experiences a natural shift occurs in his classes from intellectual discussions to how to lead an honorable and decent life. Coles believes that the roots and key to an honorable life lie in the stories learned form parents, teachers, mentors, and literature. In *The Call of Stories* (1989) he discusses the power that stories have in shaping people's lives and "testifies to the nourishing moral insights that come from narratives, beginning with stories read aloud in the family circle, and continuing through formal education and thereafter." He found as a psychiatrist, he could reach people's lives through their stories, but first he had to learn how to listen.

Coles tells of his mentor, William Carlos Williams, taking him on house calls to learn how to listen to the patient's stories. He recalls another teacher saying to him, the people who come to see us bring us their stories. They hope they tell them well enough so that we understand the truth of their lives. They hope we know how to interpret their stories correctly. We have to remember that what we hear is their story. Coles appreciatively notes that the mentors most helpful to him were those who understood *his story*.

Is there a fallacy of understanding? Is it ever possible to be so objective as not to interpret the client's story without the influences of our own stories? On the other hand, are the stories told by the clients the true story or is it the truth of the moment? What part does selective listening, selective telling, and selective memory play in the stories told and understood? They may not be precisely the event as it happened, but rather our recollections and polishing, not reality, but partially an invention.

While Coles does not deal conceptually with family stories, in telling the stories of others he is telling the story of himself and at times of his childhood. We might wonder, are the stories the family tells about itself just a way to record its history, or do they serve other purposes? These stories, according to Langellier and Peterson (1994), are often a form of social control. The story of how Mom met Dad, the courtship, the struggles; how an uncle was a hero in the war; how grandma crossed the mountains in a covered wagon, suggest ways of being, and often are aimed at giving direction. Rarely do our parents want us to find out about the skeletons in the closet.

> . . . family storytelling describes a multileveled strategic process constrained by social and historical conditions, oriented by a variety of narrative means and structures, framed by interactional dynamics of telling and audiencing, and punctuated by particular choices and actions. This multileveled strategic process functions to produce "family as a small-group culture." (p. 73)

In an analysis of family stories the authors also note how women's stories told by women frequently differ from the stories told by males. Carol Gilligan writes extensively on this topic in her book *In a Different Voice* (Gilligan, 1982). She explains that Kolberg's evidence about the level of morality is based on male "research subjects" and that morality frequently focused on logical themes and did not take into account relationship themes.

A person's life can be seen as a series of stories in chronological order. Often they highlight experiences such as birth, kindergarten, high school, marriage, death of a family member, a new job, a firing, and so forth. These stand out as special themes, perhaps chapters in a person's life. Included in these chapters are paragraphs, experiences that make up the total "landscape" of the person's life. Some experiences are remembered, most are forgotten, some are positive, and some are traumatic. Some of these incidents, for example, physical or sexual abuse as a child, play important functions in the person's development and may shape his/her life significantly. Others, such as going to the movies with friends, is just another activity and may have no major influence, yet the memories are positive and resurface when asked by a worker to discuss the fun things remembered as a teenager. It may have played an important role in building a support group of old friends or in the development of a hobby.

Similar experiences may impact persons differently depending on cultural norms or historical perceptions. Being ignored by a waitress may be seen as just poor service by a white couple, and as racism by an African-American couple. An African-American colleague tells of flying on a small commuter plane. He was the last to board and was asked to "sit in the back of the plane." Many thoughts came to mind and when he was about to protest, the hostess added, since there were just a few people flying, they had to disperse people to balance the plane. Having your suggestions ignored at a staff meeting may mean one thing to a male and another to a female who frequently experiences her male colleague's ideas accepted as the same ones that she had presented earlier and had been rejected. These are complex issues, and of course individuals usually react in ways that reduce their painful feelings, but at times they may waver from the learned, safe patterns, often at great risk to themselves.

STORIES WE COULD LIVE WITHOUT

Some stories people are told or learn about themselves are oppressive. They lead the person to believe that they are dumb, inferior, or misfits. Some are historical artifacts carried from the centuries of racism, sexism, and ethnic hatred. Stories you may know include stories of Blacks as inferior, Jews as "Gutter People" or dirty, Irish as drunkards, women as hysterical and inferior, and Gays and Lesbians as "abominations." van Dijk (1994) points out that,

> . . . typically stories about minorities usually have an overall *negative* evaluation. Positive, remarkable, events involving minority groups, are less used as occasions for story telling by prejudiced white people. . . . In other words, stories about minorities are often stories about *whites as (self-defined) victims* of minority group members or of ethnic relations in general. (van Dijk, pp. 126–127)

Anecdotal stories are used as evidence that the minority is indeed inferior, dangerous, a welfare cheat, or taking our jobs away.

These stories reflect beliefs about people and shape how they are treated by those who hold those beliefs, but perhaps worse yet, shape the way the maligned see themselves. Sometimes they come to believe the things said about themselves; sometimes they believe they will not be given fair treatment. At times, those who are discriminated against attempt to modify their lives so as to be seen as "different" than *their* group. They hope not to be linked to their group and stigmatized. This self-rejection can also lead to self-hatred and a shattered life.

No matter how persons try to cope with the oppressive cloak placed on them, negative narratives start to create negative self-images which creates problems for human development. Any group or person not treated with respect and dignity suffers in some way. Michael White believed that many of the clients he worked with came because of the oppressive or damaging narrative they had accepted of themselves. The worker can help the client to reach for the parts of their stories that reflect the person's strengths and the strengths of their group. Some groups attempt to develop strategies to deal with institutionalized and historical oppression that may or may not succeed. The "Black is Beautiful" movement was a successful attempt to combat the negative image that many African-Americans, particularly children, heard and accepted.

Children's identification with white dolls, rather then black, can be taken as an example of self-destructive decisions. It was a significant factor presented by the psychologist Kenneth Clark, and was considered in the decision declaring unconstitutional the separate but equal provisions in Southern schools, by the Supreme Court, in *Brown v. the Board of Education.*

In the mental health profession, particularly psychology and psychiatry, the work of Pavlov and Freud can be seen as leading to drastic innovations in the field. The movement of psychologists from the study of head sizes, bumps, intelligence levels, and learning theories, to counseling, was an important shift from the laboratory to the community. We might think of these paradigms as metaphors, ways of thinking about things that link to one concept and compare it to another, perhaps more familiar. Thus, the metaphor most identified with Pavlov is training and automatic response. The themes in Freud's work led some commentators to see him as viewing the person as a machine which has broken down or is in need of improving a certain part such as a weak ego. Some helping approaches see therapy as a repair shop; some see therapy as conversations; some see therapy as a puzzle to be solved or investigated; some see therapy as a series of changing stories which can be reconstructed.

Similarly, there are contrasting theories which parallel the nature-nurture dispute. Is the person most influenced by genetic factors or by social forces and learned behavior? Are certain illnesses more related to genetics, some more related to environment? What is the balance? Recent developments in plotting the genome have changed many views and will enhance our understanding of the relationship of nature and nurture. In the helping professions there are origins of problem debates. Is the problem within the person or is the problem caused by social forces or the environment? While there is consensus among most helpers that both internal and external forces are at work, the degree to which one or the other is more important has led to extreme differences in the therapeutic approaches, extending from behavior modification to existential approaches, to helping. Narrative therapy's traditional theme that "The Person is Not The Problem, the Problem is the Problem" (White and Epston, 1990) presses home the idea that it is the social context that is the major factor in fostering the concerns that have led the person to seek help. Like many of the helping approaches, claims of success are yet to be proven.

In the physical sciences certain theories and approaches are valued more highly or hold privileged positions in the field. This was certainly true for the work of Einstein, Newton, and the developers of nuclear energy, interplanetary travel, and computers. But at one time, the earth as center of the universe held a privileged position and the world as flat held a privileged position. Those who differed were laughed at, scorned, excommunicated, jailed, or worse.

In the helping field we are faced with similar situations. Certain approaches to helping have held a privileged position. Psychoanalysis, behavior modification, and cognitive therapies all have at one time or another held privileged positions in our fields. Some still do. Certainly the reason should be that they are effective and to some degree that is true, but there are other reasons as well. Just as the March of Dimes, which had been the major force behind Polio research, decided to continue and adopt another illness in order to remain a viable organization, many organizations have economic and at times political reasons to continue. Certain approaches to helping which are no longer as successful as once claimed continue to be the treatments of choice.

Historically, Alcoholics Anonymous was considered a highly successful program. High success rates, if not perfect, at least in the 70–80% range were claimed. As a result of impartial research some are suggesting the rates are closer to 30%. Similar follow-up evaluations of other helping approaches reflect similar declines in the success rates over time. This is due in part to research by more objective researchers, but may also be related to the fact that the practitioners are different. The first results usually claimed are by the charismatic originators of the programs. There may also be a placebo effect in that the status of being able to say you were helped by Freud, or by Jung, may have curative possibilities. In fact, recent medical evidence claims that placebos can in some circumstances be effective (*New York Times,* 2000).

Any new program has the problem of acceptance and exposure. New approaches to therapy are initiated in the face of entranced individuals and groups committed to certain approaches because they believe in them and have a personal and/or economic investment. To question its continued relevance is to question's one's lifetime of work. While in the "hard" sciences claims for success can be challenged and quickly tested by colleagues, such approaches are more difficult to test in the human services. It is a field where the complexity of persons and the complexity of the workers' own culturally shaped approaches make comparative work difficult. Interpretations of the problem and of success are often subjective, and influenced by one's orientation (Heineman, 1981).

For example, a mother who is on welfare survives on a minimal amount of money, raises her children, gets the kids off to school each day, helps them with their homework, and keeps them out of trouble. Is this a lazy welfare sponge, or a heroine who deserves recognition for the difficulties she has overcome? Should she be compared with another mother in similar circumstances unable to handle the situation? Who should be condemned? Even if they are the same age, and the children are the same ages, how many other variables might be at work? Does welfare create dependency? There are people on both sides of this question, and research supporting each position. Each reader might question the results of research if it came up with a view contrary to their beliefs. "What the thinker thinks, the searcher will find." People often make decisions based not on facts but on feelings. Even agreement on what is scientific research is open to question and attack with some saying only quantitative research is "real" research, while others proclaim the value of qualitative research.

These arguments in both practice and academic settings often dictate acceptable and legitimate approaches. At the time of this writing, the psychology profession is in a rancorous discourse on whether any helping approach that has not been proven to work should be supported among practitioners. Of course, this could not only influence who might practice and be licensed, but any innovative attempts to develop new treatment approaches.

These battles are not new. Foucault's work on language, power, and control exemplified his beliefs that those in a position of power often try to "subjugate knowledge." This can be done by presenting material in a foreign language (such was previously done by having religious rituals and physician's prescriptions in Latin), having a special jargon such as the DSM (Gains, 1992), and keeping groups away from materials or ideas as was done for many years to women who were kept out of colleges. It can be done by not permitting people to learn to read, as was done to the slaves in the United States.

STORIES AS METAPHORS

The idea of using a metaphor to help people understand some of the dynamics of human behavior is not new in the helping profession. When Freud talked of Narcissism or the Oedipus complex he was using stories and myths that were well known at the time and which he believed would help people understand what he was trying to say (Spence, 1984). He also used the stories that were narrated to him from dreams to help uncover the unconscious and some of the mechanisms that these dreams revealed about the person's neurosis or problem. Metaphors have been used in more general ways to illustrate the human conditions; the path of life, being at a crossroads, climb every mountain, have all been used to illustrate a challenge an individual may be faced with, or choices that people need to make at certain points in their lives. Biblical references to the shepherds and flocks is a metaphor for religious leadership. Metaphors for therapists have included friend, mentor, guru, leader, parent, priest, magician, and healer, in addition to their own titles of doctor, psychologist, social worker, counselor, therapist, and so on. There have been negative metaphors as well, "the-rapist," do-gooder, shrink, and so on. In narrative practice the metaphor might be assistant or co-author, since the helping metaphor is related to the person re-authoring or rewriting the story in their life that has brought them for help.

The value of the narrative metaphor is that stories can be rewritten, there are subplots, no client ever tells the whole story, there is always more, there are always untold experiences, that might be helpful. There are chapters; when one closes, another can begin. In addition, stories are meant to be told, to be read, and to be listened to. This suggests that other people need to be involved in the helping process. Other than personal diaries, people telling stories want and need someone to listen—it is a natural process, and a process that can be understood by clients. The stories are lived experiences, they are not theoretical; they can be examined, and they can be rewritten, often with a happier ending.

3

The Stories That Shape
Our Profession and Its Future

I am certain that my fellow Americans expect that on my induction into the Presidency I will address them with a candor and a decision which the present situation of our Nation impels. . . . This great Nation will endure as it has endured, will revive and will prosper. So let me assert my firm belief that the only thing we have to fear is fear itself . . .

(Franklin D. Roosevelt, Inaugural Address. March 4, 1933)

Once I built a railroad
Made it run, made it race against time.
Once I built a railroad
Now it's done
Brother, can you spare a dime?

Excerpt, Brother Can You Spare A Dime (1932)
Music: Lay Gorney, Lyrics: E. Y. Harburg
From, *New Americana* (Broadway Review)

Humanitarian: A person concerned with human welfare; A person advocating or practicing human action; A person believing in the primary importance of the advancement or welfare of the human race. **Humanitarianism:** humanitarian principles or practice.

THE LANDSCAPE OF SOCIAL WORK

The history of social work did not start with the Great Depression of the 1920s. Its roots are in all the religious institutions for helping the poor and needy, to the formation of hospices, to the English poor laws, to the development of charity organization societies, to mutual aid associations, settlement houses, and the establishment of asylums to house the mentally ill, just to name a few. It is a broad and deep landscape, and its story has been told and retold, and we will not attempt to tell the story in detail (Cohen, 1958; Devine, 1922; Lubove, 1965; Woodroofe, 1962). We will start our story with the era that we believe most shaped modern social work and its emergence as a major institution in our society.

Inherent in social work's historical purpose is its commitment to social justice and the betterment of social arrangements and individual effectiveness.

In an introduction to a National Association of Social Workers (NASW) code of ethics it was proclaimed that:

> Social work is based on humanitarian, democratic ideals. Professional social workers are dedicated to service for the welfare of mankind, to the disciplined use of a recognized body of knowledge about human beings and their interactions, and the marshalling of community resources to promote the well being of all without discrimination. (NASW)

The profession has struggled to explicate and translate into practice its primary concern to develop among its members three practice capabilities: (1) improve persons' quality of life and social relationships through the development of individual and community well being, competence, and mutual responsibility; (2) effectively support individuality, cultural integrity, diversity, equality, and social justice; and (3) secure the social environmental modifications and institutional supports in keeping with such developmental efforts.

The struggle to achieve these ends, that is, to create a unifying practice methodology that would allow the profession to accomplish this very complex mission and its contract with society is ongoing. The story of how the profession came to accept such a multifaceted social contract offers some clues as to the reasons it has been unable to unify itself and develop an overarching methodology.

It was not until 1910 that the census listed *social work* as one of its work categories. But that recognition, that had exhilarated social workers, quickly lost its luster and value when social work failed in its efforts for recognition as a scientific profession. The Flexner report given at the National Conference of Charities and Correction (1915) concluded that social work was not a profession. It held that it did not have its own body of knowledge and lacked educationally communicable techniques. Abraham Flexner, an educational reformer who had helped reorganize the medical profession, declared that social work's function was integrative, and that it had no standing as an independent profession (Flexner, 1915, pp. 576–590). The report both discouraged and mobilized the social work field.

The early 1920s was an era of frenzied activity aimed at making social work "scientific" and professional. Aiding in these efforts was the expanding labor market. Many middle class women were entering the labor market seeking positions that befit their standing. Social work offered such an opportunity and in 1930 the answer to "Is Social Work a profession?" was "Yes" according to Jane, or "Miss Case Worker," a character created by author Hazel Newton. . . . And "professionalism meant they were going scientific" (Walkowitz, 1999, p. 87).

World War I and the Great Depression (1929–1942) ironically led to the growth of social work. Social work education began in the early 1900s and expanded during World War I. The war's moral, social, economic, and psychological effect on soldiers and families gave impetus to the need for trained social workers. Some funding for training was made available from groups such as the Red Cross and this in turn led to the increase in educational programs in social work.

Despite the tireless work of politicians, social welfare leaders, and social reformers to wrest crumbs of welfare legislation from state and federal governments, the catalyst which enabled Social Security and Public Housing legislation to receive a public hearing and the ultimate support for its enactment was the "Great Depression."

The hurdle from the heights of economic well-being and "easy come, easy go" philosophy of 1929, to the down and out "Brother, Can You Spare A Dime" destitution of the early 1930s, was a quick plunge which left millions of people unemployed, homeless, and hungry. The unemployment rate went from 3.2% in 1929 to a high of 24% in 1933. It then started downward but remained above 9% until the war economy and army mobilization reduced unemployment rates in 1942.

Prior to the depression, the responsibility for relief and charity was clearly seen as that of local governments and private charities. But the spirit of "rugged individualism," "Social Darwinism," and laissez-faire began to evaporate as poverty spread quickly among the various strata of society.

The great economic depression began to shift the political perspective from local and private responsibility for the economic welfare of its community to the federal government; an idea that had been taboo prior to that time. This expansion of the federal government coupled with state responsibility for public welfare led to an increased labor market requiring a large number of administrators and line workers to carry out the mandated laws. The depression, a painful and, considered by some, dangerous time in our country, led to extremely high unemployment, poverty, and dislocated transient citizens who wandered the countryside looking for employment and the means to survive. The foment created by the depression radicalized many portions of the population; the government, fearful of the move toward socialist ideas, responded with social programs and the Social Security Act of 1936. Employment programs such as the WPA (Work Programs Administration) and Federal Work projects as well as the Civilian Conservation Corps (CCC) served youth and provided work for the unemployed. The WPA murals still can be seen in public buildings. Although unions had provided funds for subsidized housing, the first federal public housing was not funded until 1937.

In the depression years just prior to World War II, the radical members in the profession, the most verbal, gave social work the appearance of being a fairly radical profession. Yet there had not been a strong emphasis on federal support for social welfare or social change. Social work was as subject to the cultural/societal influences of the times as was the rest of society. Charity was a private affair in the minds of social welfare workers, as it was in the minds of other citizens. There were exceptions, such as the social work union movement in the New York area, and the work of Jane Addams and the women of Hull House in Chicago. The views shifted, however, with increasing unemployment, poverty, political unrest, and the inability of the private agencies to meet the growing demands for help. The need for government intervention became a demand throughout the United States. Under Herbert Hoover's presidency, the lack of an economic structural response to the depression led the country and its people into deeper depression. President Hoover, influenced by the historical traditions of his time, believed government intervention was outside the tradition of the American heritage. Welfare and social insurance were considered European programs and not in the traditions of rugged individualism. His refusal to take action was an important factor leading to his defeat in the next presidential election.

The newly elected president, President Roosevelt (FDR), broke with the past, and broadened the role of government in welfare. His programs highlighted a major change in the political orientation of the country, increasing the central role of the Federal government and its responsibility for the general welfare. Her biographers suggest that Eleanor Roosevelt, his wife, who had been a volunteer for many years in a New York settlement house and a strong advocate for the poor and minorities, used her influence with the President to promote many welfare programs. She later became very active in the United Nations and a leader in the fight for human rights.

While the pros and cons of the role of government in welfare discourse continues to this day, there is no longer much of a debate that certain aspects of welfare are within the purview of the government. Both Social Security and Medicare, programs mainly serving the aged, are "sacred cows," and to threaten these programs by either party means political suicide. Whether the social legislation of that time was an attempt to "cool out," and mediate the threat of radical political movements, or a moral and humane effort by a government for its people, or an effort to revitalize the economy is still under debate. It may have been all those things, but the programs aided the economy, and moderated unemployment to some degree. While high unemployment continued until 1942, our entrance into World War II, and the beginnings of the "welfare state," a name originally used to refer to the English welfare system, radically changed the institutional structures of the United States society. Were those developments important factors for the growth of social work, or to be more blunt, was it good for social work? The answer is yes!

Reflecting the profession's ongoing search for its identity and recognition, Grace Coyle, the preeminent advocate for social group work, argued that social work was applied social sciences (Coyle, 1958). Her ideas, considerably longsighted for the 1950s, tried to connect knowledge from the social sciences as the base for social work. This was an important and understandable position, as it was a strong response to the earlier Flexner report. If social work did not have its own body of knowledge, then one can argue that since social work's focus was human and social development, and the understanding of human behavior, and since the social sciences generated such research, then social work practice ought to emerge from knowledge in sociology and psychology. This had an impact on its ties to its religious roots and it separated itself more decisively from a religious orientation.

From our perspective, social work's desire for acceptance interfered in its forging ahead in the discovery of knowledge grounded in its own experiences. Flexner was still partially correct, since social work still sought knowledge outside its own body of experience for its professional knowledge base. And yet its experience and knowledge base grew exponentially, for it was privileged to benefit from the knowledge of actually working with people, rather than researching people. Indeed it was this action orientation which hindered efforts to research some of the practice that was taking place, and few practitioners systematically researched their "cases."

Social work has emphasized a contextual framework, a major contribution in understanding the behaviors and relations of persons in the environment, and extended the thinking of sociology and psychology. It has not, however, developed a social work-grounded knowledge of and approach to practice. Most of the research has been selectively evaluative, did this program succeed or fail with persons? Rarely have we asked what theories of practice are most effective. Our research questions tend more toward explanations of human behavior, and the effectiveness of programs, without singling out the aspects of practice that may have made the program succeed or fail.

Of course social workers realize that external social forces impact their clients and the agencies in which they work. But they frequently neglect assessing how as workers, they are personally impacted by those same social forces that influence their clients. In *Narrative Therapy*, Michael White (1994) maintains that all helping actions are political and that helpers are subject to the influences of social forces, the same as everyone else. The theoretical underpinnings of narrative practice stress that professions such as social work, psychiatry, and psychology are subject to the same social/political forces as clients. It is impossible to grow up in a culture or milieu without being influenced by it; no matter how much self-understanding and awareness we may have, our stories are shaped by society. Part of the professionals' self-understanding in narrative practice, is to accept the logic of that position. Furthermore it is important to realize that counseling is a political process, and subject to political social forces. Try as one might, it is impossible to be a part of society and not be influenced by the cultural influences, the media, the value system that pervades that society, as they work at being objective. It is essential for sensitive practice that social workers understand the pressures placed on them and the profession's development. Knowing the profession's narrative more fully, we may come to understand the forces shaping us, as well as what we must do to evolve into *the* profession we thought we were supposed to be, or want to be.

Our acceptance and understanding of the power social forces have had in shaping our profession and practice links us more closely to understanding that our clients are shaped by the social forces as well. We are all in the same boat, partners in trying to influence the institutions that shape us, so that we can share in a more just society. In this sense, both client and worker are shapers of society. We need each other, not only to meet our mutual goals, but to modify actions of institutions that impact our lives. *Reflection: How important would it be to the client to share this idea with them? How would it influence their self-image?*

SOCIAL WORK: HUMANITARIANISM IN ACTION

The stories that shape social work are of two kinds; they are stories of *need,* and stories of *response.* They have not been narratives of *prevention.* The narratives of *need* preceded the evolution of the profession. They are stories of the poor, of abandoned children, of people begging and living in the streets. They are stories of oppression, of illness, and of immigrants in search of work and housing. They are the stories of persons who needed support, who were lonely, persons with mental illness. They are stories that reveal people's lack of hope, and the lack of support and caring, and harsh treatment by those in positions of authority and power. They are stories of persons who demanded fair treatment and sought for ways to survive. They are the stories of persons of all ages, ethnicities, cultural backgrounds, physical abilities, genders, and economic status. They are stories of dreams denied, of opportunities denied, and often of help denied.

They are the stories great authors have written about through the ages, perhaps best exemplified by the stories of Dickens, and the vision of poor children roaming the streets of London. (And often with no ghost around to raise the conscience of the powerful.) They are the stories of people rotting in filthy prisons and institutions, which gave rise to insane asylums. They are the stories of the *"Das Narren Schyff,"* the ship of fools (see Figure 3.1). Another time and place, where people who were considered insane were loaded onto ships to be sent down river to the next town, but often dumped over the side.

The stories of beggars roaming the countryside, "hobos" riding the rails during the depression, and of bread lines, and the stories of the homeless in our own times. These stories have been written, and some have had a dramatic impact on society, forcing aloof power structures to modify the policies of neglect, at times to avoid unwanted disturbances from those

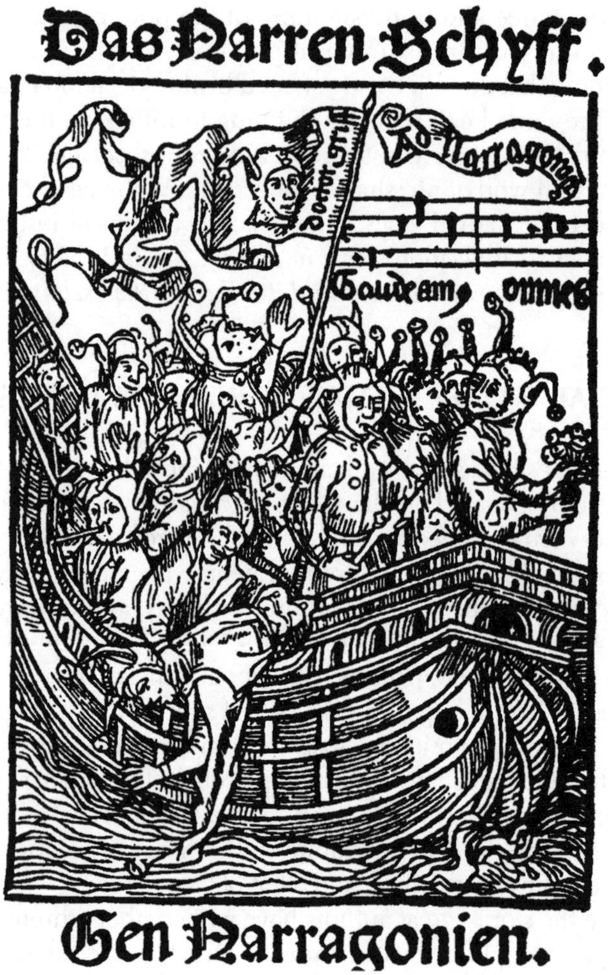

FIGURE 3.1   The Ship of Fools. A 17th century woodcut.

neglected. These stories might be portrayed in works of fiction, such as *The Grapes of Wrath,* or in accounts based on scholarly research such as Michael Harrington's *Poverty in America.* But they are also the stories of how people show the resilience necessary to continue.

The *stories of response* include the efforts of people over the years to deal with the issues raised by the stories of need, and to find ways both on an individual level and by the evolution of laws, policies, and programs to respond. These stories are often affiliated with famous and infamous names, concepts, and labels, such as "The English Poor laws," Less Eligibility, The Social Security Act, Jane Addams, Aid to Dependent Children, Settlement Houses, Friendly Visitors, the Charity Organization Society, the National Association of Social Work, the National Conference on Charities and Corrections, Bertha Reynolds, Public Housing, and countless other laws, institutions, policies, and people. They still are being rewritten by agencies such as the Salvation Army, Alcoholics Anonymous, the Y's, churches, missions, the Red Cross, community centers, family service agencies, safe houses, treatment centers, and the boys and girls clubs. All of these institutions, individuals, and concepts fit under the general category of Social Welfare, and many of those connected with social welfare are social workers. These are people who are not only educated in social work, but also persons who identify themselves as social workers. In this text, we will use that term to encompass all of those who see themselves as part of the field. It is unclear when the term "social work" was first used; it was known as "charity" work or "philanthropic work" until the end of the 19th century. The first reference to the term social work we found was by Robert Woods in 1894. "I do not wish however to differentiate the work of the university settlement too strongly from other forms of social work." Warner (1894) titled his book *American Characteristics and Social Work*, and Woods used it again as the title of an article, *Social work a new profession* (1905).

While there is now a recognition of the importance of professional education for social work the stories of some of the caregivers in support groups are as intense and effective as are the stories of helpers in agencies with degrees and substantial training. We are not suggesting that the "professionalization" of the field was not an important step, but rather that there is a great deal of important help being carried out by nonprofessional paid and volunteer workers. Their stories are important and have always been. While we recently celebrated one hundred years of professional social work, clearly, most of our basic historic "heroes" and "heroines" were not professionally trained. They were dedicated and willing to learn by experience, plus whatever more formal training was available at the time. Those early welfare leaders who did have college background came with religious training, or from a background in economics. In fact, many of the first teachers in social work did not themselves have formal social work education. They created the curriculum and the texts. They wrote the stories of social work. The first schools of social work began at the end of the 19th century. Who were the first teachers?

Some of our early narratives had greater influence in shaping the profession than others. Mary Richmond's influence enabled the growth of the Charity Organization Societies and promoted a systematized structure for casework. Jane Addams was the catalyst in the United States for the Settlement movement. The Social Security Act of 1936 was probably the key that opened the door to the major expansion in the use of social workers in state and federal government. Its initiation established federal programs that required large numbers of professionals. Since that time, major funding in both income transfers and social services has come from federal and state programs of various kinds, from public housing to health care, mental health, child welfare, and services for the elderly.

Within the grand narratives are other stories, some merely subplots, some major, such as immigration, which gave an important focus to the evolution of the Settlement movement beginning in the 1890s. That movement, along with camping and recreation, aided in the growth of social group work and community organization, while at the same time friendly visitors dealt with individual betterment, through individual "counseling," proclaiming their slogan, "Not alms, but a friend."

Slum clearance, the need for housing, the growth of highways through cities, all are "grand" stories which shaped the landscape of our country, and led to growth and jobs, but also to situations of displacement and stress. Movement to the large cities, crowded conditions, differing cultural demands, primitive health conditions, and poverty led people into agencies, which sought to help these persons adapt and make sense of their lives. Jane Addams' opening of Hull House is part of the narrative: serving immigrants, teaching English, day care, health programs, the establishment of the Juvenile Justice system, the first kindergartens, child welfare laws, and social action groups on behalf of women. The stories of the friendly rivalry between Mary Richman and the Charity Organization versus Jane Addams and the Settlement movement. The story of the Abbot sisters, whose tireless works prevented the destruction of the Social Security Act before it could become law. While almost all of the welfare was provided by private charities and a few relief programs, the great depression so inundated the agencies with people needing help that only government intervention could provide some of the help needed.

There are stories of the conflict between those interested in slum clearance, mainly social workers and social activists, and those promoting public housing, mostly planners. There are stories of neighborhood settlements opposing the building of public housing in their communities. Not all of the social welfare programs were supported by social workers.

They were often in conflict over whether the government should be involved in "charity." Some of the settlement leaders were opposed to slum clearance or public housing, because they believed, first, that some of the neighborhood would be torn down, and second, that certain "undesirable" groups would move in who would change the nature of their community. While from our perspective, now, we can see they were unwittingly supporting a segregated society, they believed they were protecting and representing the community. It is both a problem and a positive that issues such as slum clearance, public housing, and neighborhood preservation saw social workers working for agencies with one point of view, opposing other agencies with another point of view, often equally rational and moral from their agency's vision and mission.

In those early days, it was not expected that social workers would have social work degrees; most of those working for social welfare in the thirties did not. They included Jane Addams and the Abbot sisters, one of whom became the dean at the school of Social Work at the University of Chicago. Non-social workers often led initiatives for what we now see as important welfare services. The story of Ernest Bohn rushing by overnight train from Cleveland to Washington, D.C. as soon as he heard about the passage of laws providing funds for public housing is a narrative reflecting his foresight and concern for persons. It provided some of the first public housing in the nation, and made Cleveland a model for housing advocacy under the new laws. We will never know all of the stories of our profession, and its many allies and enemies either for that matter. Buried in the minutes of many agencies' board meetings are references reflecting discriminatory actions, for example, to deny the building of public housing, or halfway houses in their communities. Not only was there fear of the stranger, or the minority, but the desire to maintain the community's culture.

Even during World War II, when factories in industrial cities were importing workers, many areas of the city of Cleveland, for example, would not provide temporary housing for "Negroes." While social workers often fought for integration, the problem was often the laws that protected segregation, including covenants in housing sales, preventing sales to minorities. We may never know many of the profession's stories. We often were just too busy to write. We may never know, for example, the story of who first coined the term social work. It may forever remain a mystery.

At times social work's stories simply parallel the story of America—the movement west, the growth of new towns and cities, the use of immigrant labor, the rust belt, the war effort, the civil rights movement, the demands of women for equal treatment, the "coming out" of gays and lesbians. Some of these stories reveal the context in which our profession functions and establish our belief that as a profession, we cannot help but be influenced by the political/social forces of the times. Perhaps a low point in our profession's history was the dismissal of Bertha Reynolds from her teaching position at Smith College because of her "radical" political views, and her attacks on McCarthyism. Her inability to find employment in social work, at a time when there was a vast shortage, is evidence of our own profession's subjugation by the political context. All of these are stories that have shaped our profession, created needs, and created responses. Our response was to evolve into a profession which dean Nathan Cohen proudly described as *Humanism in Action* (Cohen, 1958).

> Social work today has found a methodology and a two-pronged approach growing out of the two types of humanitarian influence. The two-pronged approach includes concern, on the one hand, for the adjustment and development of the individual toward more satisfying human relations and, on the other, for improving the social institutions within which the individual functions. (p. 8)

One of the key figures in bringing new direction to the practice of social work and attempting to integrate the two-pronged approach was William Schwartz. He might very well have been one of the first post-modernists in our profession. Although his major background was in groups, he introduced new concepts into the social work perspective, breaking away from those he considered false. In his seminal article, presented at the National Conference on Social Welfare in 1961, he made a strong case for developing a generic practice framework that crossed the boundaries of individual, group, and community practice. He maintained that the function of the worker was to mediate the process through which the person and society reach out for each other in a common search, through mutual aid. His proposed five universal social work tasks to be undertaken by every worker no matter the particular area of practice—whether group, family, individual, community, or organization. They are:

1. The establishing of a contract between worker and client around what is to be done;
2. Challenging the obstacles to working on the contracted tasks;
3. Lending a vision as to what might be accomplished;

4. Searching out the common ground. (Particularly important in a group and community setting. It has implications for the nature of the relationship between worker and client in all settings.);
5. Giving information to the clients to help them make goal-directed decisions, the giving of knowledge.

Schwartz's approach, the "interaction" or "mediating" model, was immediately accepted in social group work, and subsequently, but more slowly, made inroads into the general social work field. In that same article he explained the importance of systems thinking. While systems had been introduced earlier by Gordon Hearn, it was not generally accepted into social work until the late 1960s. Realizing systems theory was too static, and did not take the contextual environment into consideration, it was picked up and expanded into systems and ecosystems approaches by both Carol Meyer (1976) and Carole Germain (1981). At about the same time, in a jointly authored book, Germain and Alex Gitterman (1980) promoted both the ecosystems and the interaction perspectives.

Social work's stories are still being written, and re-authored, partly because it is a profession in search of a practice theory, and a dynamic profession, constantly responding to the demands of a society which itself is in search of equity and justice. While it is no secret that many of the approaches to helping it incorporates are derived from other professions, particularly psychology, it is also no secret that there is a great deal of injustice, which social work sees as its mandate to counteract.

New laws and policies are emerging which reflect the demands of minority groups. Racism and homophobia are stories of the ongoing struggle for social justice. The conservative backlash against welfare programs has led to time-limited service, placing women and children into dire poverty, without adequate food, health care, and housing. While it has cut the welfare roles, there is uncertainty as to its success in the long run.

Within the profession itself there is conflict between those dedicated to the nonprofit public social services arena, and the growth and impact of managed care and private practice. Particularly troublesome to a profession whose roots have been in the public arena, this movement is seen as traitorous to some, a disregard for our mission, and paradoxically as a step toward status and growth, and professional recognition. There is some concern that those in private practice do not identify with the profession. For example, many list themselves as "psychotherapists" and not as social workers in the yellow pages of the phone book.

In addition, our profession's story includes subplots involving the stories about marriage and family counselors who compete for many of the social work positions. There are the stories of the nurses, who have taken over social work positions in hospitals, particularly in discharge planning. While there is an increased demand for social workers, and an increasing number of social workers are entering the field, the membership in the National Association of Social Work is declining. Their annual national conferences have been suspended and replaced by local meetings that primarily focus on continuing education courses (CED) for licensing credits, rather than the presentation and sharing of new ideas.

Part of social work's story has been subjugated; that is, it has been neglected and hidden from view. A major example is social work's contribution in the area of family therapy. Nichols and Schwartz (1998) write

> No history of family therapy would be complete without mentioning the enormous contribution of social workers and their tradition of public service. Since the beginning of the profession social workers have been concerned with the family, both as the critical social unit and as the focus of intervention. . . . Indeed, the core paradigm of social work—treating the person-in-the-environment—anticipated family therapy's ecological approach long before systems theory was introduced. (p. 24)

They then go on to explain ways in which contributions of social work have become subjugated.

> That the importance of social workers and their ideas have been shamefully underemphasized in the history of family therapy says something about how opinions are formed in our field. Social caseworkers have been less visible than the trendsetters in family therapy because they have been busy, working in the trenches and delivering service, rather than in academia, writing books and making speeches. (p. 25)

There may be other factors as well, a major one, the gender issues. They write, ". . . the orthopsychiatry movement which helped define the landscape of family therapy, was dominated by psychiatrists, who grudgingly recognized psychologists, but devalued social workers and their contributions. Why this historical lack of respect for the profession of social work? One reason might be that "the early social caseworkers were mostly women writing for a field primarily populated by women. . . ." (p. 25). Their work was subjugated, ignored because they were women and their work was not privileged.

We might add that narrative practice is undergoing a similar subjugated process in the social work profession. Jane Gorman notes, "By devaluing narrative as a method of understanding and change, the scientific ethos in social work has repressed a powerful mechanism of societal consciousness-raising and change" (Gorman, 1993, p. 247). The Council on Social Work Education on a number of occasions has turned down papers related to narrative on the basis that it is "not relevant" to the profession.

A major evolving story within our profession, one that is shaping our direction, is related to the growth of private practice and the increasing move into the predominantly clinical or therapeutic arena by social workers. While our historic stories have always included both the emphases on individual and social change (see NASW statement), there is growing evidence that there is movement to the therapeutic. There are a number of reasons for this drift, some outside the control of the profession. These include who and what insurance companies will reimburse for service, the status of doing "therapy," and the independence it gives the professional. Related to these are the nature of the demands of the social agency setting. Large welfare departments have been bogged down with rules, paperwork, and large caseloads. These factors have led to some agencies reflecting an assembly line model, rather than a caring institution.

> A former director of New York's Department of Social Services, and a graduate of the Harvard Business School said, "I visualize the department as a big paper factory . . . you put the client on the conveyer belt at the beginning and she gets off at the other end with a check or some other service. Social workers are fine . . . but these are problems that need real resources, real teeth. It's the biggest data processing show in town." (Abels, 1973)

One other point that may be an important factor is that the clients in these agencies are often looked down on, seen as lesser persons, attacked in press and TV, and some of those working with them want to disassociate themselves from that context. If in addition they are not treated with respect and dignity by the agency administration, when they have a choice they leave such agencies, many setting up private practices, or moving into private practice on a part-time basis.

There are countless stories, which reflect the evolution of the social work profession, and while our profession's stories are multifaceted, they reflect two major tracks. The first, with roots in the charity organizations' societies, led to casework, and the therapeutic; the second were the efforts at social change, which evolved into work with groups, community organization, and policy development. These are most often identified with settlement houses and community planning agencies. While it might very well have been rational to evolve into two separate professions, the leadership in the 1940s and 1950s saw it as a necessity to maintain one professional direction. While this idea has created the unique profession we have become, we have been in an ongoing quest to find the theoretical base that could unify the disparate practice and often philosophical differences that the two functions, the therapeutic and social change, require. Social work has not been able to develop a practice that easily encompasses the complexity that social workers deal with every day. A mother on Welfare may need funds, she may need counseling, and she may need the kind of supports which a nonexistent program might provide. In addition her child may need medical care and a day care program. The social worker might legitimately be expected to deal with all these areas of need. The variety of knowledge and skills needed to deal with clients in such multi-problem and multi-need areas are awesome and illusive.

The establishment of a unified social work organization in 1955 was an effort to merge the various nonprofit social work professional organizations into one umbrella organization, like the American Medical Association. Under the leadership of Chauncey Alexander, who was its executive Director, this worked well for a number of years. During the civil rights movement in the late 1960s the Association for Black Social Workers was formed. The group workers formed their own organization in the late 1970s, and the clinical social workers started their own organization at about the same time. Each felt that their interests were not being met sufficiently. The National Association of Social Work in 1995, facing this splintering movement, started subprofessional groups with which specialists, such as alcohol/drug and school social workers, could align. So they too have started to aid in the fragmentation, while hoping to keep these disparate groups under one umbrella.

The Council of Social Work Education has also tried to maintain the salience of a single profession by insisting that to be accredited the schools of social work teach a generalist framework, that is, the student would be exposed to learning practice with systems of various size from individual, groups, family, and community. They could learn specialized areas after their introduction to a generalist perspective. This has certainly exposed the student to the range of practice in the profession, but there is a question as to whether the impact carries any further than mere exposure.

Surveys of incoming students indicate a growing number, often a majority, saying they intend to enter private practice as soon as they get their license. There may even be a larger percentage by the time they finish their education. After seeing the treatment, and caseloads of social workers in state child welfare departments, and assessing the status given to "therapy" by both their fellow students, faculty, and the community of social workers, they can't wait to do their time so that they can get their license to practice "Privately." Part of the rush to private practice is a result of the profession's efforts to be recognized as a profession. It pushed for licensing, a worthy idea, but with sometimes disastrous consequences. Some states only license "clinical" practitioners. We are then faced with unlicensed agency executives, who although they may have years of experience can not supervise new MSW's who are seeking credited work hours for their own license. Agencies spend money that could go for services to clients, to pay for supervisors who are licensed, so that new social work graduates would be willing to come to work for them. In that way, they can get required supervised hours by a licensed social worker. In effect, in some states clinical social workers have come to dominate the profession, and push it in their desired direction. This too has led to a fragmented profession. We do not see narrative as a solution to these problems. It is a concern that only the major professional organization can handle, if it wishes. But it does support the theoretical underpinnings of narrative which point out how power structures shape the professions.

Clearly, however, one of the major problems facing our profession is that there is difficulty in developing an approach to practice which encompasses approaches of individual and social change within its practice theory, philosophy, and practice techniques. It is this quest for a unifying approach to our profession that led us to the narrative practice landscape that emerged out of what has come to be called the postmodern era.

THE CURRENT SCENE: POSTMODERN AND CONSTRUCTIVE APPROACHES IN SOCIAL WORK

One of the strengths of social work is that it is always searching for alternative approaches to practice that will increase its ability to serve. It is not tied too closely to any one theory, since most of them evolved external to the profession. Ann Weick in discussing reconstruction in social work noted:

The bridge to the development of an alternative view is based on a constructive approach, which assumes that processes of human knowing are
deeply rooted in and shaped by our culture, conditions, and psyches.
Because perception itself if mediated by constellations of factors, the possibility of seeing something "as it really is" is no longer tenable. (Weick,
1993, p. 170)

The postmodern, constructive approaches in the helping professions
owe much of their development to the feminist and civil rights movements. They helped, sometimes forced, society look at cherished beliefs,
myths, and policies that tend to keep people in subjugation. While in
the social sciences the initial attacks were on the White-Male Power
Structure, the postmodernism movement began in literature and the arts.
It then moved into the psychological and social sciences literature. In
brief the "modernists" were searching for a scientific paradigm to explain
life forces and to make therapy more scientific. Theirs was a positivistic
approach, searching for the one truth to provide the answers. The postmodernists question whether such a truth exists, seeing them as social
constructions, subject to complex internal and external forces, including
political power.

Freud was seen as one of the first modernists. He was attempting to use
science to explain human behavior, and was instrumental in changing
our understanding of behavior, and of treatment in mental health. The
postmodernists have questioned some of the "science" of Freud and the
directions that modernist approaches have taken. The questioners see
the modernists as interested in control and power, as directive experts.
They have seen the modernists in therapy as insensitive, or unaware of
the needs of women and minorities, and neither reflective nor appropriate in their helping approaches. While this is certainly an overly broad,
and partially unsubstantiated attack, there is no doubt that there are
some approaches which have become privileged, in that they are taught
in schools, or promoted by workshops and books, even though evidence
of their success is sketchy. Postmodernists seek to explore other models,
suggesting that none should have precedence over others, unless proven
better. They maintain that there is no one "true" way as to how people
should be helped.

Joan Laird, one of the authors who has written broadly on the postmodern movement in social work, is an advocate of Narrative Therapy.
She edited a volume of articles on social work and the social constructionist approach (Laird, 1993). Her introduction reviews the growing

postmodern, constructivist influences on our profession. She points out the earlier social workers who questioned the positivistic, scientific paradigms, noting the work of Martha Heineman in 1981, and the early questioning of "scientism." She notes the evolution of a group that began meeting at CSWE meetings, and evolved into "The Study Group for Philosophical Issues." They have put out a newsletter and have presented a number of papers at conferences. She points out that,

> It wasn't until the late 1980s, however, that the field began moving in any major way beyond a critical stance, beyond a deconstruction of prevailing doctrines toward what are becoming major reformulation of approaches to research, theory and practice in the profession. And it was the early 1990s before a re-visioning of social work education entered the realm of possibility. (Laird, 1993, p. 3)

Her introduction also examines the differences between modernist and postmodern approaches to practice, and the collection of articles are theoretical and practice-focused.

The constructive approaches have been taken up by other social work practitioners and educators. Gorman, a social work educator, advocates for a social work approach that incorporates postmodern approaches and presents an important review of the evolution of postmodernism as it impacts our profession, comparing it to the modernist philosophies. She points out the movement from positivist research and the quest for a "grand theory" to an approach that reflects our profession's humanistic approach (Gorman, 1993).

Anderson (1999), a therapist who has been involved in postmodern therapies, particularly narrative practice, notes,

> A postmodern-social construction perspective invites self-reflection on our traditional beliefs, including those on the family and family therapy. It invites multiple voices, diversity, and differences; it invites collaborative relationships; it invites vitality and excitement back into our profession; and it invites connection and response to broader cultural contexts and issues. (p. 7)

Constructivism is closely aligned with Narrative because it focuses on how people create meaning in their lives, Brower points out that this is clearly seen in group work. Partly as the group members begin to, ". . . develop a shared understanding of the treatment setting" (Brower, 1996, p. 336). This requires them to be in an open place in which the group begins to become more cohesive, and meanings are shared. What does

Brower mean by being in the right place? They must have the language, concepts, and awareness. Some see this awareness as part of the ecosystems approach.

What are Constructivist Techniques?

How do we use stories to make sense of events, to find meaning? Clients are questioned about themselves, talking, as they will about their lives. In essence, the clients tell us the story of their life. Not just the story of the problem, but highlights, memorable happy and sad events, their visions and hopes that they had for themselves as they grew up. Those are the visions they hope to achieve. Thus they are involved in their life landscape, viewing its beginning, present, and hoped for future. Their future story is yet to be written and will be with the help of the worker.

Denins Saleeby (1994) states, that, "Professional social work can be substantially enriched by incorporating constructivist appreciations and perspectives into its theory and practice. To do so may require a shift in our understanding of the nature of reality and our stance toward what is 'true'" (p. 351). He includes the works of Epston and White noting their statements. He emphasizes that the quest for "meaning" is an important part of practice, pointing out that there is an emphasis in the helping professions to move from the idea of problem to solutions. Saleeby references de Shazer (de Shazer, 1982), who maintains that clients must be involved in "creating scenarios of possibility so they move in directions more satisfying to them" (Saleeby, p. 357). In a narrative mode, White might use the concept of "re-authoring" as a means of helping the client achieve the same results.

We believe that narrative practice gives us both the philosophical/theoretical base and the techniques that are syntonic with the historical culture of our profession. It provides both the intellectual foundations and vitality that can unite the field. Narrative goes beyond the traditional helping techniques by incorporating social change and individual resistance and protest within its theoretical and practice philosophy. By doing this it carries out the historic mission of the profession. The breadth of narrative's approach and creativity makes it particularly valuable and appropriate to the field of social work, a profession committed to individual and social change, and to social justice. While it assumes the therapeutic stance, it is therapy in the broad sense of change, rather than solely individual healing.

THE NARRATIVISTS IN SOCIAL WORK

At the time of this writing Narrative Therapy is still mainly the domain of the Marriage and Family Therapists, even though Michael While clearly identifies himself as a social worker. Part of the reason for this was that social work's extensive history and experience made it more difficult for new ideas to penetrate the mainstream of the profession. Marriage and Family Counseling, on the other hand, as fairly new areas of helping, was seeking something it could latch onto and claim as its own. It became an area of interest and White was quickly called upon to lecture on his work, mainly to non-social work audiences.

A number of training videos, based on live client interviews, were made by the Pace Institute in Los Angeles, a private educational institution which has become a major training ground for marriage and family counselors in the California area. During the period of the 1990s, only two social work agencies in the Los Angeles area were using narrative extensively. While there has been some increased interest, mainly due to a few narrative therapists, and the course developed by P. Abels at Cal State, Long Beach, it is still facing an uphill battle. Clearly there is increased interest by the social work community and a number of articles and training programs have came on the scene to greet the new millenium (Hartman, Laird, Abels). In 1997, Kilpatrick and Holland, in a book on social work with families, inserted a chapter on Narrative Therapy. This has tended to increase the exposure, since it became a text in courses dealing with family social work (Kilpatrick & Holland, 1995).

Continuing her work on constructionist thinking, Laird in 1995 wrote,

> the postmodern movement in its various forms, constructivism, deconstruction, poststructuralism and social constructionism, is generating new thought and theory in the arts and humanities . . . In social constructionist thought, knowledge is not some measure of reality separate from either the knower or the process of knowing . . . Human knowledge is subjective, that is a matter of interpretation. (pp. 150–151)

She openly connects constructivism with Narrative Therapy, when she points out that,

> Epston and White . . . argue that problems should not be located inside people or even in their relationship between people. People have problems because they and/or others have or are making sense of (or authoring) their life experiences in ways that inhibit their moving forward and consequently

are disempowering. In other words, the experience itself is not the problem, but rather the narrative describing the experience. In these authors' view, people have problems with problems, change occurs when the relationship between the person and the "problem" evolves. (Epston & White, 1992, pp. 153–154)

In an interview for *Reflections: Narratives of Professional Helping*, done by Joshua Miller (1999), Ann Hartman discusses her interest in Narrative Therapy:

J. M.: Tell me about your travel plans.

A. H.: We are traveling to Sidney for a few days and then to Adelaide, Australia, where Michael White's family therapy center, the Dulwich Center, is having a narrative family conference. Joan (Laird) and I will be doing a one day workshop on the social construction of gender and sexuality before the conference and then repeating an abbreviated version of this at the conference. We are also leading a brief discussion with other educators and supervisors on the pros and cons of the teacher in the classroom adopting a transparent position. After that we are going to Kangaroo Island for three days and then we will be in a one-week, intensive small group with Michael White.

J. M.: What do you find meaningful about your work with Michael White?

A. H.: He certainly has been the person in family therapy who has been most influential for me in the last six or seven years. I think the depathologising, empowerment, and respect for clients and the recognition of their truths—all of these things are very congruent with my values and very exciting in terms of working with people. I have already been to three workshops with him in Cambridge and we have gotten to be quite good friends, so I really look forward to spending some time with him. And he is a social worker. (Miller, pp. 67–68)

THE INNOVATORS OF NARRATIVE THERAPY

A major theme of White and Epston (1990), the prime movers in Narrative Therapy, is that "the person is not the problem, the problem is the problem." This emphasis sets the tone that the person is not to blame, and that the person's situation must be examined in context. While this emphasis helps the worker remember not to put the blame on the client, it is still a narrower perspective then we would like to see. While there is no doubt a percentage of situations where clearly there is evidence that some internal, perhaps genetic condition is involved in the problem, it is our belief that most of the situations which people face that create problem situations for them are contextual and mainly social/societal. We believe as did both Mills (1959) and Schwartz (1974) that private troubles are all public problems. This is not to pardon the hardened criminal, or the drive-by shooter, but it does suggest that these events, no matter how reprehensible, must be viewed in the context of the narrative of the landscape of the person's life. Fortunately, the social worker is not required to judge the person, but to help them move to a more positive and societal acceptable life. This can be done as the person attempts to develop a story for himself/herself for the future, and one that has some reasonable chance of accomplishment. In narrative practice this is seen as a "re-authoring" process. In light of our thinking we would like to suggest that more emphasis be placed on contextual issues, and that this is a necessity if we are going to develop a more suitable social fabric which is able to develop the environment in which persons can develop in cooperative, moral, and positive creative ways. In short the development of a just society necessitates that the context is one which supports all people and treats them with respect and dignity. We therefore suggest a frame of reference, which takes as its underlying theme: *The person is not the problem, the contextual situation is the problem.*

Narrative Therapy has been on the scene since the late 1980s. Most of the initial work was done by Epston and White and appeared in various journals in Australia and a newsletter put out by the Dulwich Center in Adelaide. It was the publication of their seminal work *Narrative Approaches to Therapeutic Ends* that made their work more widely known in the United States. It is only in the past few years that it has been referred to in the social work literature. It is still not widely accepted and still unknown to most professionals. It is taught in a few schools of social work, and considered by some as not being representative enough to be presented at social work education conferences. It has gained a much wider following with the marriage and family counselors, and numerous articles related to it have appeared in Family Process, most written by family therapists.

One might ask why it has gained such wide acceptance by one group and been ignored by another. The most salient response is that the newer profession MFCC is not as wedded historically to a hundred or so year history of problem-focused approaches to helping. It has not yet hardened into a profession with a hundred years of literature, organization codes, rules, myths, and rhetoric that surround the social work profession. Social work has an entrenched reputation, which has ties to certain approaches to helping. New ideas are not incorporated easily. Certain approaches have held a privileged position in the profession's practice theology, and these approaches tend to be modernist.

The first of the modernist helping approaches to reach prominence in the United States was the Freudian, Psychoanalytic model. The Freudian structural approach became the dominant model and was emulated by much of the social work profession, particularly those who were "case workers." An alternative model, taught by the Pennsylvania School of Social Work, was based on the Rankian analytic philosophy. It was not able to compete with the Freudian landscape, and faded off the scene in the mid 1960s. Some of its contributions, particularly around the use of time, and agency function, became important and lasting contributions to the social work field. For many years the Freudian approach was seen as the predominating model, and psychoanalysis the preferred treatment approach. The influence of Skinner led to the development of behavior modification approaches, which became very popular, and became a major theoretical approach of the University of Michigan School of Social Work for many years.

Other privileged approaches have included psychodynamic approaches, gestalt therapies, and hypnosis. Almost all schools of social work attest to using systems and/or ecosystems approaches, but as it has become clear that these are not "practice" models—supporting practice therapies have been attached to the systems models. The current preferences are cognitive approaches. Following the psychological influence on our profession, the work of Beck seems to prevail as the approach most popular for individual practice. In family therapy there seems to be the widest application of different approaches, where it seems to be that new ones come on the scene each year. Almost all of the traditional models have their adherents, but many workers see themselves as eclectic, using a number of different approaches, or at least techniques from a number of approaches, if not the entire paradigm. This shopping-mall approach is likely to continue until there is strong enough evidence that one model seems to offer the most positive results. In the family therapy field, the approach which is beginning to appear most attractive is Narrative Therapy.

4

Understanding the Narrative Approach

No story is the same to us after the lapse of time:
or rather we who read it are no longer the same interpreters.

George Eliot

Client: A person who employs the services of a legal adviser; a person whose cause an advocate pleads. A person using the services of any professional; a customer. A person assisted by a social worker.

(Oxford English Dictionary)

All persons are concerned about the future and, to varying degrees, they make decisions and take current actions based on their hopes for the future. To that extent, we are all futurists (Abels, 1977b). A bright spot in human evolution is the realization, certainly in this new century, that people can increase the control of their environment and their future. Our greatest disillusionment is the growing feeling of hopelessness resulting from having done it poorly and having lost control. For those seeking ways to regain a sense of direction for themselves and for those they care about, narrative helping offers a way to do this that is empowering and self-directed, and respectful.

Narrative practice is rooted in the philosophical orientation of the postmodern constructivist modes, which aims to help the clients maintain the direction of their lives, and minimizes the use of authority by the worker. In an article related to deconstruction, White says, " I would like to think that I have a critical constructivist or constitutionalist perspective" (White, 1995a, p. 66). Indeed, the style of his work with people is extremely affirmative.

Freedman and Combs (1996) in their text *Narrative Therapy* note,

> Using the narrative metaphor leads us to think about people's lives as stories and to work with them to experience their life stories in ways that are meaningful and fulfilling. Using the metaphor of social construction leads us to consider the ways in which every person's social, interpersonal reality has been constructed through interaction with other human beings and human institutions and to focus on the influence of social realities on the meaning of people's lives. (p. 1)

Although many therapists have adapted narrative tools such as "externalizing the problem," they remain allied with other theoretical models (McQuade, 1999). Certainly, many narrative techniques are valuable, but as White (1995a) suggests, narrative practice is more than a set of techniques—of course that should be true of any form of social practice. It is grounded within a system of belief that frames the way help is offered. There is an integrated, quasi-permanent totality to an approach and without the integration of the thinking and doing the approach is limited. It is important therefore that we look at some of the basic orientation that might allow the greatest possibility of success. He writes:

> The narrative metaphor, in conjunction with other metaphors, as a philosophy of working with people, are commonly used in family therapy literature and practice—specifically metaphors of system and pattern. It is very often assumed that the narrative metaphor can be tacked on to these other metaphors, and the narrative metaphor is often conflated with them. Because the metaphors of system and pattern on the one hand, and the metaphor of narrative on the other, are located in distinct and different traditions of thought, this tacking on and conflation of disparate metaphors simply does not work and in my view, suggests a lack of awareness of the basic premises and the very different political consequences that are associated with these different metaphors. (White, p. 214)

There are three areas of concern. First, the importance of the practitioner's worldview relative to the success of the narrative approach, a view that expects the worker to recognize the importance of context and the social forces that impinge on persons. Helping is dependent on treating persons with respect and dignity, and in fact, caring about the person. Respect does not mean admiration, but rather respect for the person as a human being in and for him/herself. It accepts the important principle that the person's narrative is the person's own story. The worker disallows his/her own learned therapy narrative to impose on the client's story, and works to be honest to him/her own self; neither to impose or place a masked narrative on the client. For example, a client might explain that he keeps hearing voices and he is frightened by them—and the worker might interpret, using his/her own narrative perspective: "Yes I'm sure it's frightening but the voices are not real, even though you might feel that way." Here the worker places his/her own social reality on the client as a context for the unembodied voices. These voices have no context, yet to the person they appear to speak with authority and objectivity. The narrative practitioner might help the client by aiding them in deconstructing the content, the structure, and the meaning of the experience. He/she might ask questions such as "What are these voices trying to convince you of at this time? What are they trying to talk you into? How do they fit in with plans for your life? Are the voices supportive or controlling? Are these voices in favor of you having your own opinion and knowing what you want, or are they against your opinion? Are the voices helpful in clarifying what you want or your direction? Who do these voices remind you of? The confusion these voices create is in the service of the voices, not in the service of the clients. How can the client be helped to gain control of them? The worker would be working closely with the medical persons involved with the client and would not suggest the client not use their medications.

The worker's values encompass respect for all persons, a willingness to listen and learn, and a belief, transmitted to the client, that the worker is not all-powerful. The sources of knowledge required for change to take place lie within the person's impetus to access and discover in his/her own and others' life experiences. These may evolve from views of other workers during a reflecting team discussion, suggestions from people with similar experience, and such sources of knowing as books, stories, art, music, friends, family, and other endowed entities.

Second, it calls for the worker to accept that there is new knowledge, often unique to the individual and/or group, that needs to be learned in order for narrative practice to be a helpful process for the client. Since it is client-related, contextual knowledge, we can often do little more than support some of the efforts being made, and reflect on some of the social work guidelines present in the profession since its early history. These "knowledges" take into account what clients seek and the impinging social forces. Knowledge is needed on how to help particular clients make connections with others, and how to design structures that create opportunities for persons to make those connections. Narrativists suggest that the worker take a "know nothing" view. The worker's biases need to be set aside, and furthermore, since each client is an individual, we really know very little about the meaning of this helping experience for this particular client.

The third major area is for the enhancement of the skills that make the re-authoring process possible. These skills are enmeshed in a philosophical framework that recognizes that techniques alone do not suffice in the helping situation. It is necessary that a relationship occurs in which the client believes not in the worker's power, but in the worker's concerns and efforts to help them be their own person. Skills of relationship building are based on mutual respect and the client's deeply felt belief that the worker cares about him or her. This calls for a relationship of mutual respect where the clients are aided to discover and gain their own competence and remain in control of finding their own way—a relationship of respect and shared vision of how the future might be shaped as they share the tasks necessary for the re-authoring process.

A WORLD VIEW FOR NARRATIVE PRACTICE

The person's world view is a set of fundamental beliefs, attitudes, values, and knowledge that influence a person's comprehensive outlook on life. The fundamental sources for this outlook come from all aspects of a person's life including culture, family, peers, gender, religion, sexual orientation, location, economics, and life experiences. It evolves into a frame of reference that organizes the person's perceptions of others and the world in general.

> There is a dominant story about what it means to be a person of moral worth in our culture. This is a story that emphasizes self-possession, self-containment, self-actualization, and so on. These notions are seen to be specifying or describing a way of being and thinking that shapes what is referred to as "individuality." This individuality is a way of being that is actually a culturally preferred way of being. And what is "right" is culture specific. What's "right" requires certain operations on our lives, much of which are gender and class-specific. (White, 1995a, p.16)

This world view forms the responses one might expect from that person on a fairly regular basis; it helps distinguish one group from another. A world view is part of what makes a particular group a different group. It can set the parameters for what people accept as the truth, and provide a structure that limits and/or expands the pathways for those with that world view. Culture, gender, age, economic standing, and ethnicity all have something to do with a group's world view, but that does not infer that all persons share the same world view because they are of a certain age, socioeconomic class, men, women, cross gender, or other. Culture and language shape thinking because they affect the meaning persons give to their life experiences. Education influences persons' world view, and as they learn other views, their own traditional values may be modified as they reflect on and experience others. Education is a marvelous instrument of change. Frequently the purpose of education has been to tap into human inquisitiveness, to encourage intellectual doubt when disagreement occurs among reasonable persons, and to search for "truth" as best as it can be known.

Postmodernism and constructivist approaches influence the world view of most narrative therapists. Modernism, an outgrowth of the enlightenment, sought decisions based on science and rational thought (Gergan, 1985). This perspective influenced most social work research with a confident emphasis that social work must have an empirical base. That truth could be scientifically known is a positivist approach to science counting more often on the results of quantitative research than qualitative. Postmodernists do not reject research and the need for empirical knowledge. Rather they reject the notion that one truth for all persons can be found, particularly within the social sciences. In the social sciences there are so many variables, there is no objective reality waiting to be discovered. Societies and cultures are fluid and knowledge changes over time. As economic hierarchical societies developed, even within a democratic context, we recognize that certain persons and beliefs held a privileged place in the society, resulting from an unequal distribution of power, and the control of knowledge by those in a position to do so (Foucault, 1965, 1980).

We are informed that persons create their own realities and that reality is subjective. But we also know that reality is created in relationship with others, and the concept of "the individual" often ignores the process through which a person becomes who he/she is; this depends on their experiences as member of a family, a group, a classroom, a committee, and the multitude of significant contacts and attachments made in their life narrative.

THE SKILLS OF NARRATIVE

Recalling some of the items we discussed in earlier chapters will help us gain a fuller understanding of narrative practice. Basic, of course, is to recognize that a person's life is made up of bits and pieces of experiences that we have called the "landscape of their life." These are put together in ways that help the person make sense of his/her life. Out of countless personal experiences many are forgotten but some are deeply recalled. Some are good, some horrid and better off forgotten. From that landscape of experiences, particular incidents are influential and powerfully instrumental in directing the current movement of the person or the person's family to seek assistance. While these events are catalytic, part of what the worker knows (their knowledges) is that there are many unrevealed subplots in the person's life, beyond the story being told. The worker deals with the immediate narrative, and the variations, additions, and omissions are responded to as the process unfolds. Over time, other pieces exposed as factors amplify the problem situation, uncover and establish the person's strengths, and often provide clues that help clients re-author their lives.

BEGINNING

Workers are familiar with the difficulty people face in making decisions as to whether to seek help or not. Previous disastrous helping experiences and/or their historical autobiography makes help seeking seem inappropriate. How does one make that first experience less stressful? Certainly it is important to treat the client with respect and to make them as comfortable as possible in the strange setting they are about to enter. Jay Haley noted that at the start of a first meeting, clients should be treated as you might welcome guests in your home (Haley, 1971).

The narrativists frame the meeting as a conversation. It is a *conversation with a purpose*, a purpose helpful to the client. The conversational mode means that a minimal number of personal questions are asked at a first meeting. We suggest that the orienting idea might be, what is the least amount of information I need to be helpful. There is no end to how much data can be found out about a person. In some settings, such as a welfare department, administrative law requires many questions, but even there the questions can be spaced over the length of the session so as not to bombard the client with a breathless series of questions. Different approaches might be used: questions are scattered throughout the meeting, explanations given as to the why of the questions, their importance, and the time taken. If notes are required, these too should be kept at a minimum and the reasons explained. It is imperative for the worker to review the questions prior to the meeting and consider putting aside those that could be answered in other ways. For some, both the client and the worker write the answers together. For example, things to be remembered, questions to be asked later, things that may not be clear are to be noted for further clarification. Agency requirements related to what is done with the material should be explained, and the right of the client to see what has been written should be discussed.

Many clients who come to a professional helper may not have experienced respectful responses, and may not have been treated as persons able to take control of their own lives. Previously, they have been told the things they must do to get better, or are told the behaviors they are required to perform. Many of the institutions in which they are involved tend to be autocratic, with many rules, an overworked staff, and a pressure to "get on with it." The conversation of mutuality creates a violation of initial expectations, that is, being treated as person when you expected further humiliation. This initial violation of the client's expectations is a valuable action. It is not meant to be manipulative, but is based on the idea that it can help the person see that this is a unique opportunity, a safe place in which there are many things that the client can say and do which would not be "acceptable" or seen as a positive "out there."

For example, a solo (single) parent bringing up children and believing herself to be worthless because of the welfare label and general abuse by uncaring systems, might be helped by looking at what she has been able to do for her children in spite of systemic indifference and by helping her see herself as a fine, caring, and productive person who has had to overcome stultifying obstacles in order to make a decent home for her children. How many people faced with the problems she has had to overcome would be able to do as well? This is a recognition of the strengths, coming out of her own life experiences, not the creation or pep talk of an authority. The structuring of the context by a relevant reflective conversation begins the re-authoring process, and enables the person to begin the work on sculpting themselves toward the future and their preferred ways of living. Much of the work of the helper is in the asking of reflective questions and in helping the person examine the roots of some of their beliefs, helping the person see the contextual factors involved in the presenting problem.

EXTERNALIZATION OF THE PROBLEM

A basic artifact of the narrative approach introduced by White and Epston is the process of *externalizing the problem*, a process that has

caught the fancy of helpers from many different perspectives. Externalization modifies the internal conversations persons have about how bad
they are, how much they failed, how ugly or unworthy they might be. It
moves their internal conversations into more positive and productive
thoughts by helping them to find an external force to focus their change
efforts. Nichols and Schwartz (1998) note, "From the outset, the problem is seen as separate from people and is influencing them—'it brought
them there' . . . the therapist's questions about the identified problem
immediately imply that it isn't possessed by anyone, but instead is trying
to possess them" (pp. 410–411).

In their book on Narrative Therapy, Epston and White present a situation illustrating their work with a six-year-old boy who suffered from
encopresis (White & Epston, 1990, pp. 43–44). This work was influential
in establishing the unique character of Narrative Therapy. It highlighted
new ways of looking at helping, and raised considerable interest. The
therapist in the situation helped the young boy examine the possibility
that "sneaky poo" was an external force influencing him to do all of these
things. Together they sought to find ways to overcome the influence that
"sneaky poo" had over him. White calls this process externalization of
the problem. As we examine this concept in the context of their development of helping approaches, we see just what power exists within this
idea emphasized by the theme that *the person is not the problem, the
problem is the problem.*

White explores with the client their experiences with the problem, by
introducing "externalizing conversations." This frequently requires a shift
in the patterns persons use in thinking about themselves and their problems. It's like moving away from attaching the feeling of stupidity to yourself when you strike out in baseball. It is not unusual to find persons
engaged in internalizing conversations about that which is problematic.
This is largely a cultural phenomenon, one that so often reproduces the
very problems that persons are attempting to resolve. So, parents might
say, "Johnny's the problem." In response, White will ask questions that
introduce externalizing conversations about that which is problematic.
"How is the problem affecting Johnny's life? What is it doing to his
friendships? How is it interfering in his relationships with you as parents?
What do you think it is doing to how Johnny feels about himself as a person?" He asks Johnny some of the same questions, and this approach supports externalizing conversations (White, 1995a, p. 22).

Externalization is a technique, a philosophy, and a way of thinking
about the situation. It encourages both the client and the worker to try to

understand the experience in relation to the recent historical context, and to both the actual and potential resources available to the client. Concurrently the worker is considering the resources available. What does the agency offer that can be used? What resources is the worker aware of and what might be needed? Who else can be involved who might have additional views on what might be helpful? Are there persons who could help make important decisions? Are there persons who the client would feel comfortable having at the meeting ?

The purpose of the externalization process with clients serves to encourage persons to objectify, and at times to *personify*, the problem that the person experiences. What do we mean by this? To give the problem a name, like "anger" rather than just talking about how he/she gets angry, and how that gets him/her in trouble at school—"I just fight with other kids all the time." Then to personify "anger," by talking about how anger gets him to fight all the time. If the client says he procrastinates a great deal, to ask how "procrastination" gets him in trouble at work or at school. If the person can be helped to think in this way, and reflect on how procrastination becomes oppressive and controls his/her life, and explore the discomfort procrastination has caused, a plan may begin to evolve to overcome procrastination. It takes the self blame out of the picture. Persons, according to White, are often *problem saturated*, and if they are helped to understand they are not the problem, not to blame, and that external forces have a lot to do with what they are going through, externalization becomes a "freeing" mechanism.

In the context of this interaction the worker is pressed to think of the person in relation to the problem, and the problem in relation to the person. The interaction permeates all worker actions, and is reminiscent of the social work concept of the person as social self, or person in the environment. Externalization is not a catch phrase, but a continuing effort to emphasize the importance of the contextual as a force in the helping process.

In the case of "sneaky poo," an external enemy created and agreed upon is faced and, with serious reflection and adequate resources, dealt with. The child is not the problem, but is being acted upon by the problem, and in turns responds in certain ways, some of which he/she can achieve without "Sneaky Poo's" cooperation if he is willing to give it a try. This in no way relieves him of responsibility for what he is doing, but does say he is able to find ways to overcome the obstacles that caused so much distress. These techniques are part of the narrative process and rely on aiding the child to find aspects of his/her history to serve as levers for change.

At first, reading this perspective appears to create fantasy, rather than helping the child deal with the reality of his needing to control himself. Such questions are legitimate and important to consider. A more traditional approach might explore the underlying causes for the child's behavior. Concepts such as seeking limits, attention, control, a sense of safety, defecating on the parent and getting even, might be realistic concepts that fit some theoretical underpinnings. But we really do not know the cause. We may never find out, no matter what theoretical foundations we come from. Does creating an external force, which appears to control some of the person's behavior, take the responsibility away from the person? No, because the person still has the responsibility to find ways to change in the face of the obstacles, and or to change the obstacles, the forces that have created the situation. Does it take away the person's responsibility for their alcoholic behavior, does it suggest that in abuse and battering the perpetrator bears no responsibilities? No, it does not. It assists the person to reflect on external factors that influence the behavior and how they can alter that influence, but certainly does not condone the batterer's actions.

Reflection: White suggests that we take on a "know nothing" stance when we first begin working with a client. We are not experts on the client's problem, nor do we know the cause, or the reality of its impact. All we know is the story the client tells us, and we need to know more. We do not know the meaning the experience has for the person, or whether they will be able to mobilize the forces required for change. We want to help the child quickly overcome a condition troubling to him/her, and most assuredly to the parents. If the child was in kindergarten or first grade, "sneaky poo" may create a problem for the school, and the parents might be told to take their child out of school. The effort to uncover underlying causes would be extensive, and yet the worker is still left with helping the child cease the behavior. Of course in the example we have eliminated causal differentiations such as abuse. We know that the child could consider "sneaky poo" as punishment, or as a way to keep the abuser away from him/her. Externalizing the problem reveals those obstacles that prevent the child from overcoming or taking control. The narrative that reveals the abuse moves the worker toward a different tact. In essence this all means that the "causes" are not within the child's internal emotional makeup. They relate to the child's interaction with forms of oppression. Our professional assignment, then, in addition to the legal responsibilities, remains the same: to aid the child to be safe, and develop his/her own capacities and to seek the aid of others to prevent oppression. This approach frees the child from self-blame, creates a sense of ownership of her/himself, and involves other adults in the process of creating a safe place.

On the other hand, there are valuable benefits to the child by this externalizing approach that need to be considered. It might be that he sees that going for help could become a game that could be played. He is respected and joined by an adult interested in finding a way to trick "sneaky poo." The fact that he has to become smarter, and to watch out for his tricks, could catch the imagination of the child. In addition his parents' distress may have lessened. To stop being blamed for something, which may or may not be as annoying to him as to his parents, would be an added benefit. Of course the parents are helped to understand what the child was trying to do as he attacked the problem, and enter into the action with the same end in mind, to overcome "sneaky poo," a trickster impacting all of their lives. *Reflection: It is important to remember that children have a lot of make believe friends, and it is not too difficult to gain another. It might also be that some of his make believe friends could be called upon to work with him to defeat "sneaky poo."*

Let us leave this story for awhile, although we may return to it in time to examine other factors of relative importance to narrative and explore the idea of externalization a bit more. Earlier we spoke about how stories shape persons' lives, and how for some, stories told to them or their group may be oppressive. Clearly these orienting narratives have a strong influence on how persons see each other, and others.

CONTEXTUAL INFLUENCES

What happens if a child is brought up to believe that she/he is dumb? How many children have been ridiculed in a classroom? Do you recall that happening to you at any time? What happens when a woman is brought up to believe that she is not entitled to go to college? What happens when a group is treated over long periods of time as inferior or as outcasts? Imagine if those persons also read about themselves as inferior, and "scientists" repeatedly point this out in the media. Consider how movies portray persons in subservient roles, indicating that they are less important and less valued than others. What groups are generally depicted in such roles? What happens if people are taught that they are superior, entitled to treat women or others as inferior? People tend to believe the stories they experience as they grow up. And if, in addition, they are treated in ways that support certain class, gender, ethnicity, age, and other destructive narratives, they are more likely to accept those stories as true.

These stories of being ugly, dumb, and unentitled shape peoples' lives, just as the stories told to the Kennedys, the Bushs, and the Roosevelts about their mission to be leaders of society are absorbed and shape their lives and ambitions.

While some negative stories are not meant to harm, and are told thoughtlessly, repeated as myths, jokes, and half-truths, they still may harm. Some stories are deliberately meant to denigrate because they reflect the true feelings of one group's view of another group. For example, some attacks on gays and lesbians generally accompany stories that describe homosexuals as unholy, in violation of religious perspectives, or "family values," to be spurned, beaten, and damned to eternal hell. For example, one Roman Catholic priest who was working with gays and lesbians was prohibited from ministering to them, and was rebuked emphasizing, ". . . that homosexual acts are intrinsically disordered, and evil" (Niebuhr, 1999).

A Mormon young man, who is gay, was put out of his home by his parents and forced to leave the church. He told his friends that Mormon elders come to see him every year, wherever he might be, to persuade him to stop being gay and return to the church. On one hand, he says, the Morman church cares, and on the other hand the church does not accept him because he is gay.

A group's beliefs can have serious consequences within the context of every social institution of society, in social relations, in unequal treatment, and in physical safety. Such is certainly the case with homophobia. It has often been seen as a license by some people to be abusive and kill, even by some law officials.

Some stories are created based upon years of prejudice or because it serves those in power to retain or gain more power. The falsely created *Protocols of Zion*, which fabricated a Zionist takeover of the world, was one such story. It was used at first to get the Czarist government to oppress the Jews, and later used by the Nazis as they sought a scapegoat to enable them to gain power in Germany after World War I, and to promote "Aryan purity," or "ethnic/racial cleansing."

Settlers' desire to gain the Western lands led to the creation of many stories treating the First Nations People as bloodthirsty savages. By treating people as inferior, or less worthy, all kinds of oppressive acts can be committed against them. These stories can and have been repeated countless times, worldwide. Just change the names of the oppressed group to suit the occasion. What we are concerned with is the damage done to people when the aftermath of these incidents leaves economic, social, and psychological scars. Beyond the economic poverty, the cultural devastation inflicted, and the diminishment of access to the "good life," many persons are led to believe they are less worthy than others, evil, dumb, or less attractive. This can lead portions of society as seeing others as less civilized and less intelligent, which can lead to such behavior as the society not respecting schools that have large populations of immigrant groups, or persons of color. In turn this can result in students "dropping out." It can lead to young women not believing they are thin enough, which can lead them to become anorexic. At its worst, it leads to a country allowing genocide and apartheid as we saw in an earlier chapter. The distinctions created by such narratives violate efforts to built a just society and have been and should be a factor dealt with by the social work profession.

Some stories that groups have come to believe can become very dangerous, even when the stories are related to groups other than their own. The resistance of African-Americans to deal publicly with AIDS was due in part to past negative experiences in the health arena, particularly research related to their group such as the Tuskeegee syphilis studies. Although they have come to suffer disproportionately from the disease, very little was done by people in their community, says one African-American Reverend, because of their belief that AIDS was a gay, white male disease. One minister noted, "The attitude was 'Thank God it wasn't us.' Many churches didn't want to deal with the stigma or with drug abuse" (Brozan, 1999). On an international scale we see South African leaders resisting promoting some AIDS treatments partly because they are developed by the white power structure and not to be trusted.

Persons start to internalize stories about themselves and their group. Even when they do not accept them totally, they are harmful and can create shame and even self-hatred. Some persons in an attempt to become more "acceptable" try to take on the style of these who have attacked them, trying to look and act like them, and when possible assimilate to that more powerful group. Internalizing the problem makes the person feel that they are to blame. It leads to discouragement and often a feeling of helplessness. This can be particularly true if the group you belong to is often singled out in the media, in books, and in public discourse. Often they have no grand figures of their own from their group who can be looked up to and seen in heroic terms. In addition, many of the contributions of the group are not known or have been suppressed. The lack of certain minorities in movies or TV or in major political positions is often given as example of this neglect of diversity and of control by the power structure, which is most often seen as white and male. While there are obviously changes taking place, historical decisions make the process a slow one.

A caveat needs to be offered here before we proceed. In a way, narrative practice is a form of resiliency practice. It is known that some persons escape the effects of disrespect. It has been assumed that a factor effecting their being resilient is that as they have grown they had connections with some adult(s), generally outside their family, who have cared about them and truly respected them. In all persons' narratives, those who have not escaped the branding of the destructive stories and myths that prevent social, educational, and psychological health, there are bits and pieces within their history that have not yet been formed into their life narrative. These are experiences in which they succeeded, overcame a problem, and/or did something wonderfully kind and generous. None have been incorporated into their overall framework of living. In narrative practice the worker aids persons to discover those tucked away experiences that aid them to re-author or construct how they want to be—to find their fountains of acts of resiliency. *Reflection: Foucault speaks of subjugated knowledge as a means to keep hidden some of the contributions of a group, or in the use of certain language like Latin or psychiatric jargon becomes a means to keep knowledge secret. Since knowledge is power, this gives the controllers of the knowledge a great deal of power.*

Externalizing the problem helps persons see that the problem is not within them. While their feelings about the problem are in them, their reactions to the problem are within them and the ability to deal with the problem is within them, the cause of the problem may be contextual, that is, created by outside forces. Taking this perspective carries the notion that if change is to take place, some of the changing has to be not only the perceptions of the clients, but also their ability to understand and deal with external forces in a different way. There is a melding here of individual change and social change. While this may not be true in all cases, it occurs in most situations, such as viewing the family as a context within other contexts with which the person must deal. This is certainly true in spousal and child abuse. Okin in a discussion of women and equality in *Is Multiculturalism Bad for Women?* offers powerful evidence and an explanation of how some religious cultures violate women's individual rights of equality over group rights, creating serious abuse of women (Okin, 1999).

Externalization can often serve another purpose with the client. It can upset the traditional orientation they may have had in their life experience. A teenager who has not been getting much help from a wide range of helping and educational professionals may be astounded when asked, "Why does anorexia want to kill you?" Or to ask an alcoholic, "If Al is such a good friend of yours, why does he get you in trouble?" By placing the problem outside the person, and asking a different order of questions that make this external force "lifelike," the person is aided to think differently about the situation. Avoidance, passive listening, and profound hopelessness can be jarred by such unusual questions. It also calls for creative responses and embraces them in the externalization process. It minimizes the person's feeling that here is just another thing wrong with me, to be added to all of the other things that I have been told are wrong with me. It emphasizes the person's awareness of strengths and suggests the promise that there is a way to deal with what's going on, and that it will take work.

The more the problem can be externalized, particularly with clients who are "problem saturated," or what in social work used to be referred to as the multi-problem client or family, the stronger the hope that change will take place. For the worker-client dialogue to examine that there may be external forces that are involved in having created the situation, which the client sees as his/her problem, enhances the relationship between the client and the worker. This is a framework for understanding and work that must always remain in the worker's mind. At times, the contextual forces are so overpowering that they need an immediate response—such as a child about to be thrown out of school. The action might be an immediate call to family, discussion of what to do, an immediate call to visit the teacher or principle to explain the situation, and engaging the others (authorities, family) and, if possible, the child in seeking alternatives. Epston and White have used the writing and sending of letters to key persons in such situations.

At times it may be clear that the problem is internal to a degree and that external interventions may not be helpful. That calls for intense work with the person to help them understand that only their actions may modify the situation. That does not negate the efforts of the worker to help the person understand where their actions may have been learned, as well as aiding them in identifying experiences where their positive actions modify the situation. Work with men who abuse their wives would be one such example. Either in a group or individually, the work needs to explore the unacceptability of such actions and the sources of belief that such behavior is acceptable. It would be greatly disrespectful to try to persuade the spouse to accept such actions, as to "understand" why her husband batters her, and/or that she has any responsibility for his battering. Some theories of helping hold both parties responsible for the battering, and lend credence to therapists doing just that. Frequently situations where such "nonaction" by therapists occurs lead to continued abuse and worsening conditions for the woman being abused (White, 1995a).

Rambo, in a wonderful book on her creative therapeutic practice, tells of an interview, in which a wife and husband discuss all of the labels the husband has been given by therapists to explain his behavior. It has come to the point where the wife has come to believe she is the cause of his abusing her. At a culminating point the husband says he can't control his behavior because as the therapists have said he has . . . The therapist interrupts asking, "Have you ever hit your boss?" "Of course not," he responds, "I would be fired." At that point the wife, seeing the reality, declares, "So you can control it" (Rambo, 1993). The wife sees that he is able to control his abusive behavior if he wants to, but doesn't try to do so with her. In this situation, previous therapists became unwitting partners in the wife's continuing abuse. The revelation that the husband is able to control his temper becomes a learning experience for the wife, and changes the direction of the helping process. *Reflection: What theoretical/practice framework do you believe that previous therapists might have used with this family? What is the impact on the couple by workers putting a diagnostic label on the husband's situation?*

MAPPING THE PROBLEM

While externalization is the strong link in helping the client recognize how the "outside" impacts him or her and the problem being worked, mapping the problem addresses the connection between the problem and the person's personal contacts. In this process, the worker attempts to discover with the client and the others involved in the process how the problem impacts not only on the client, but also on those involved with the client. In the case of the little boy, clearly the mother and father are involved. Is the teacher, the boys' friends, neighbors, anyone else involved? In the above case the parents are asked to discuss how "sneaky poo" impacts their lives. This helps them to see just how they are involved, and also serves to take some of the pressure off the child. The parents are helped to externalize the problem, so as not to treat the child

as the problem, but it is "sneaky poo" who needs their attention. They then become involved in the process of trying to deal with "sneaky poo," rather than attacking the child.

The mapping of the problem also aids the worker and the client in understanding the contextual nature of the problem. Who is involved? How does the problem impact them, how do they react to it? Does their reaction create additional stress for the client? For example, do other children in the class avoid him? Does the problem keep him from staying at other children's homes overnight? Does it make his parents angry with him? These types of questions are what White refers to as *Relative Influence Questions*. He uses these questions as a means of creating a structure that supports externalization of the problem, noting, "relative influencing questioning is particularly effective in assisting persons to externalize the problem" (White & Epston, 1990, p. 42).

Similarly, a person who is drinking too much would be asked to examine what happens to him/her on the job. Does it get in the way of his/her work? Do coworkers get angry if the job doesn't get done? Do they want to go out to lunch with him or her? How does it impact his/her home life? This questioning process creates a picture, a map if you will, of how the problem impacts the overall life of the person, as well as the environment in which the person acts. This picture not only becomes a clue for the worker as to who might be involved in any helping situation, but also enables the client to become a witness, testifying to his/her own experiential impact and the systemic ramifications of the problem.

Some examples of externalizing questions on various subjects that might be used as well for mapping the problem include:

How does "worry" keep you from doing the things you would like to do?

When "frustration" gets the better of you, how does he make you feel? How do other people react to you when frustration takes over?

Does "thinness" keep you from going out with friends? How come "thinness" knows what you should eat?

UNIQUE OUTCOMES

Unique outcomes are situations that exemplify times in which the person was able to deal with the problem. For example, was there ever a time when Al (Alcohol) tried to get you to drink more and you decided not to even though you might have liked to? Can you tell me of a time you were able to go through the night without wetting your bed? What was special about that night? Was there ever a time you didn't let procrastination keep you from getting in a paper on time? Exploring these unique occasions with the person helps them to see that they do have a certain degree of control over the problem, whether it is "procrastination," "alcoholism," "the wet jet," or other externalized problems. If they are able to do it once, they can do it again. The husband not hitting his boss is such a unique experience. It would be important to ask him as well whether there were times in which he was able to control his anger at his wife. How did this occur? It is also important if there seems to be a pattern of when the person is able to exert control and when they can't. If there is a pattern, it would be important for the client to examine the conditions. There may be signals that the person can recognize that would alert him or her to approaching problematic conditions.

THE PERSON'S RELATIONSHIP
WITH THE PROBLEM

How did the person get connected to the problem? Where did the idea come from that it is ok to beat your wife? Did you learn it at home? Did his friends do it? Has he ever been part of a conversation where this behavior was generally discussed? How did the person get recruited into accepting abuse, or believing they were unworthy? While these are part of the important story-gathering which gives some clues to further action, it also serves as a way to understand how the impact of the problem on the person changes over time. Does it have as much control as it did? Does the client feel any change in the power relationship with the problem?

As the helping process evolves, it is important to examine with the client whether their relationship to the problem has changed in any way. You might simply ask if they are able to control their drinking more now than they had been before. Are they wetting the bed less frequently? Are they getting angry at work less often? Are the relationships at home better or worse? What you are trying to determine with them is whether or not they are more or less able to control the problem now that they have labeled the items they are going to work on. They then can be asked to discuss in what way the nature of that relationship has changed. The responses might be as simple as responding by giving a number: "I have only had four drinks this week on Friday on my way home from work. I usually get drunk."

The narrative practitioner might then ask whether the client thinks this is a good thing or not. In a sense the helper is asking the person to give testimony to their own ability to change and that indeed this is a good thing. In addition, the client might ask why it is a good thing, further involving the client in a reflective process.

Another way that the change in a relationship can be examined is by simply asking the client to record on a scale, from one to ten, as to how the problem influences them. Then they can be asked to do the same about how they felt when they first started the helping process or even last week. In this way comparisons can be made, and the client can see the changes as witness to their own self-evaluations. For some persons, being able to see the actual figures on a chart may have more meaning than talking about the change.

RE-AUTHORING

The narrative that the person presents to the helper is the current overpowering story, usually a negative or depressive one that brought the client in for help. It is formatted from historical experiences as well as what might be occurring in the person's life currently, a subplot, but not the desired story. The nature of the helping request is that the future be different and that the story in narrative terms be re-authored. Narrative practice is future-oriented. The goal that both the client and the worker have is to help the client consider what they would like to see for the client in the future, what is the story they want to produce, or re-author, and what story line will help them achieve that end. *Reflection: Although narrative therapists avoid the concept of contract, and see it as a power in the hands of the worker, the idea of re-authoring is in a sense looking at the goals the client hopes to achieve, and then finding the means by which these goals can be achieved.*

The worker and the client work on the preferred story that the client hopes to achieve. These stories must contain within them some series of steps in which actions aimed at dealing with the problem are discussed and adapted as the contextual situation permits. If poverty is the problem, then preferred stories might include employment opportunities, welfare opportunities, or perhaps educational opportunities that become part of the dialogue between the worker and the client. Both internal and external forces are examined by both, as the re-authoring process takes place.

As the conversation unfolds and the worker asks questions about the nature of the person's experiences, there is no attempt to press the client into any predetermined step-by-step process. While the worker needs to know why the person has sought help, and what areas of concern she/he may want to deal with, the process is conversational and reflects the client's storytelling manner. Workers at times are concerned about clients' verbal abilities and willingness to talk. How does that influence the nature of the conversation? There seems to be some evidence that when the interview is more like a conversation than a traditional interview the client is more able to talk about their problems in a relaxed manner. They do not feel that they have to respond to a series of questions often on a long form or checklist.

This may be a problem in some agencies where the traditions and/or policies of the agency require the filling out of long "intake" forms. Even in such situations, however, it is possible to scatter the questions around some of the meeting rather than dealing with them all at the start of the session. In some cases that initial questioning, particularly in a welfare department office, can take up most, if not the entire, first meeting. This in itself can be a very discouraging factor in creating the kind of helping relationship the client is hoping for.

Relationship is a key factor in the belief on the part of the client that the sessions are meaningful, and that they have been helped. We might even point out that to this point in time there is very little evidence that any one model of helping is generally more successful or effective than any other. There is evidence, however, that the nature of the relationship does impact the client's view as to whether they were helped or not.

LETTER WRITING TO CLIENTS

A unique approach in narrative practice is the writing of letters to clients following a session. We will devote a chapter to this interesting and effective technique later in the book, but would just like to say a few words about it here in this compendium of narrative. Rather than keeping extensive records, the worker may send a letter to the client informing them of some of the thoughts the worker had during and following the session. These letters often include positives that the client needs to think about, such as, I was interested in how you got the insight as to some of the troubles "hate" involved you in. You seemed to have more control of "hate" at our last meeting; had anything occurred that gave you added control? Workers maintain brief notes of the sessions.

om Anderson, who has made use of the reflecting team in a number
ays, some different from White's, discusses how he uses it with clients:

e generally meet with new clients for consultation to get a picture of the
uation. This consultation usually takes from one to three sessions. I say
e" because, if it's acceptable to you, we like to work as a team for this
nsultation. What we generally do is have a therapist meet with you and
terview you. This interview is observed by one of three colleagues who
e actually watching and listening to the meeting in another room
hind a one-way mirror. They do not talk behind the mirror. At some
int in the interview you and your therapist will change places with
em. For example, if I were meeting with you, after about forty minutes
u and your family (husband/wife/mother/child) and I would go into the
her room and my colleagues would come into our room. We would
en watch and listen as they discuss their ideas about your situation and
fer suggestions about how to proceed in the future.
   After they finish, which is usually in about five to ten minutes, we will go
ick into the room, and they will return to the other room. We then talk
out their ideas and see which of them, if any, seem useful to you.
   The purpose of this method is to generate as many ideas about your sit-
ation as possible, including how to address the issues and what to do
garding future conversations and meetings. Does this sound acceptable
you? (Anderson, p.110)

lichael White has a variation in the use of the team. It is usually a
p of from four to six people, and they discuss the strengths that they
in the conversation that takes place between the worker and the
it. It is less of an assessment and prognosis, and is used more as a
parative and supportive device.

CLIENT AND WORKER RELATIONSHIP

re is a great deal of research which supports the view that the nature of
relationship between the worker and the client accounts for most
e change that takes place in the therapeutic situation. Regardless of
method used, the relationship holds a major role in the change
ess. Narrative practice recognizes this important factor and empha-
that the client is the worker's best consultant as to what needs to done.
getting started with the client, White points out that he wants to
out what life is really like for the client.

Some agencies are concerned about having contac
writing, other than official notifications of appointment:
terminate, and so forth. During the first time I taught n;
one of my students wrote a client, on his own. When tl
out, they called the school's field department liaison to fi
letter writing was all about. They were concerned with tl
tions. It led to a session on narrative with over a hundred
In addition, I informed all students from that point on 1
the narrative techniques without discussing them first
agency. In addition to letters, narrativists often use logs, c
and co-writing with clients (Bacigalupe, 1996).

THE REFLECTING TEAM

Most of us are familiar with one-way mirrors, whether thi
edge of their use in agency practice, or from police ai
movies in which the person is being observed for their
ments. It was used quite extensively by the Milan school o:
ily for the therapists to discuss the clients situation with e;
course of the practice. At times, the client was privy to the
Anderson (1991) started to use it in his work with clie
observing group would also present a critique of the proce:
White and Epston (1990) have made this a mainst;
The reflecting team is trained to examine the client's stai
portive manner. They talk about their own experiences i
the experiences that the client has had. They raise ques
talk about what the client or the worker should be doii
are no negative reference at all in any of the tapes that I
rative reflecting teams at work.
The reflecting team serves three major purposes. Fi
support group for the client by promoting the person's (
Second, it provides feedback and points out similar expe
well the client has handled them. And third, it serves
expertness of the worker.
The way White and Epston use the reflective experi
client to react to the comments. This gives the client a
discover that others see value in the way the client has h
tion. It also provides them an opportunity to become ;
own interactions.

So, I guess the first part of my work is to try to get some appreciation of what persons have been going through. I think that it is important that I achieve a degree of understanding about this, and I think that it is important that persons are aware that I have achieved at least a degree of understanding. (White, 1995a, p. 21)

This is a way in which both parties in the conversation begin to gain confidence in each other and start to see each other as partners to the encounter.

An important part of the building of a relationship with a client is related to a fundamental concept in the social work approach to helping. That is, that all people are to be treated with respect and dignity. White's view of successful therapy reflects this principle.

I'm really interested in what persons determine to be preferred ways of living and interacting with themselves and each other. . . . If the ways of living and thinking that persons often come into therapy with aren't working for them, for whatever reason, I'm interested in providing a context that contributes to the exploration of other ways of living and thinking. There is always a stock of alternative stories about how life might be other versions of life as lived.

He goes on to point out that at times he must join in challenging the structures that dominate peoples' lives and make change difficult. "So at times, this practice of therapy includes a form of political action at what we might call the local level" (White, 1995a, p. 19). *Reflection: Revisit the purposes of social work as described in our history. Have we had approaches similar to narrative therapy? What would some of our early theorists think about narrative?*

In the course of working with clients, a number of incidents discussed will be particularly offensive, the abuse of women and children, the putting of lye in an infant's bottle, and so forth. While these are clearly offensive acts, not to be condoned or honored in any way, the worker needs to explore with the client the meaning of the experience to him/her within a social context This may be difficult to do in the face of an openly cruel and disturbing situation, but if the client is to move to preferred stories these connections need to be made.

Narrative practice involves the use of the clients' life stories as a means of helping them understand how the problem has come to influence their lives. It holds that the problem is external and not within the person and ways can be found to overcome the problem. It assists the person in looking at the context, how the problem may have latched on to the client, and influences his/her life as well as others connected to the person. It then helps the person re-author his/her narrative and work for a preferred future.

5

Doing Narrative Practice

"From today you are all crazy."

(Orphanage in Canada)

Doing: action, conduct, performance. Effort put into accomplishing something.

(OED)

A CONVERSATION WITH A PURPOSE

When does it make sense to go for help? Of course, some people have no choice. They may be institutionalized, mandated by the courts, or children. They have no choice. Some of the persons we have had conversations with or about include the boys who called themselves Batman and Superman. They had no choice in whether or not they would go to the mental health center, but their parents did. In talking with the parents we found that some wanted their children to have contacts with children their own age; some wanted their children to do better in school. All of them tried to make sense of the situation. Some had hopes that their child would become "normal." They all felt some guilt about the situation. They were all trying to make sense of the situation, and since bringing and picking up their child every Saturday morning was a major commitment, seeking help called for careful consideration.

Then there was Sam, a young man about 30, who was concerned because his fiancée had told him she would not marry him unless he got some help. A college graduate, he had lost 3 jobs in the past year. Now employed as a shoe salesman, he might lose this job as well because he was beginning to lose his temper too often with the customers.

Or Mrs. L., whose child was going to need kidney dialysis, and was urged to join a support group with other parents whose children were also going through similar treatment. There could just as well have been a support group for the children too.

Roger, a Vietnam veteran, expressed constant guilt about the war. He had nightmares and, unable to sleep, was constantly in a rage and drinking heavily. He had been to a number of therapists. The last one urged him to get involved in a veterans social action group. He wondered if it would be any better than the Alcoholics Anonymous group he had attended for awhile and then left.

There are others who come to mind. A physically handicapped teenage girl who tried to commit suicide because "no boy would ever love her." A tenant who had lived in public housing about 30 years, and had seen her mother raped there. Prisoners, who just wanted someone to talk to. There were many parents who were concerned about the problems their children were having in school or with drugs. Some had a choice and others did not. All were anxious about the new experience; some hoped things could be better; and some had no hope at all or at least they said so.

Before people come for help they are faced with trying to make sense of the decision to do so. The stories that have gotten them to the point of deciding to do something different about their lives start to be modified or adjusted to account for the need for an outsider to help them. The ability to make sense of, to find meaning in, the experience that they are about to enter, is an important part of the process. It will be determined in part by their gender. Women are more likely to see help-seeking as acceptable. It will be decided by their cultural milieu. Some cultural groups resist going outside their group because it may be shameful or alien to their beliefs. Some groups or individuals may forbid persons going for help, particularly if they are women. Sometimes, perceived external dangers may keep certain groups from seeking help from the "outside," for example, gypsies, First Nations persons, people fearful of the "authorities" like undocumented aliens; those who see institutions as dangerous, that is, a place where people take your children away. For many of these people going for help does not make sense because their experience or their "group" has taught them it is not acceptable or too dangerous.

It is important for the worker to realize what a major undertaking requesting help may be for all persons, and particularly for those who for whatever reasons have learned it may be a questionable action. While the vast majority of agencies provide sensitive, respectful, and effective services, there are some that are more concerned with secondary gains or their own welfare than ensuring the welfare of those they serve.

One of the most harmful examples of agencies disregarding the damage to clients occurred in an agency serving orphans in Quebec. "On March 18, 1954, the nuns came in and said, From now on you are all crazy. Everyone started to cry, even the nuns." Thus reported Herve Bertrand of Canada. He was one of 3000 children living in 12 orphanages in Quebec which the Roman Catholic Church transformed into mental hospitals in the 1940s and 1950s to reap more generous government subsidies. The agencies could get three times more to care for a mentally ill patient than for an orphan, so they declared the children mentally unstable or retarded (Farley, 2000). This report in the *Los Angeles Times* certainly reflects an unusual incident, but the consequences for the children was devastating and lifelong. There is evidence of other agencies treating various groups in discriminating ways, and reports of fraud in billings by agencies are well documented. See, for example, how clients most in need are often assigned workers with the least amount of experience (Lorber & Satow, 1977).

Most people who resist going for help do so for other reasons than fear of the agency. In an individualistic-oriented culture, it is difficult to admit that one needs outsiders, a stranger, in order to feel better about yourself, and that you can't handle your own problems or make a better life. No matter how trivial the concern might appear to the helper, for many people it raises fears, internal debates, doubts, and for some a major attack on the person's self-worth.

The account of what brings them to the worker will often be a construction, which illustrates the turbulence they face and which has gone beyond their usual abilities to cope. Other than for those who are mandated to go for help, persons must believe that it will make sense to seek help. While they try to find some meaning in the situation, they also ponder what the meaning of going for help will be. Help-seeking must make sense according to the context of their own personal experiences and historical development. The person must find some personal meaning, either embedded in the landscape of their real life experiences or in a sense of hope for the future.

The lack of ability to make sense out of a situation can lead to the type of action or inaction that can have devastating impact on the person. In his classic article, "The Loss of Sensemaking in Organizations," K. E. Weick (1993) reviews the incident in which a number of fire jumpers lost their lives, in part due to not being able to make sense of a situation. Surrounded by a fire which they could no longer control or easily escape from, they were facing death. The team leader, who they did not know very well, shouted for them to drop their tools and burn the area surrounding them. Faced with a command that made no sense to them, they did not and ran, most to be burned to death. The leader who had burned the ground around him survived. Weick pointed out some of the reasons the men refused to listen — one was their lack of personal experience with the situation and the leader; one of the most important reasons was that they did not yet trust him, and what he told them did not make sense to them (K. E. Weick, 1993).

> When people can no longer find meaning in their situation — whether because some crucial attachment which gave purpose to life has been lost or because the interpretive structure has been overwhelmed by events it cannot grasp or contradictions it cannot resolve — the loss of any basis for action causes intense anxiety and searching, from which new meanings has to evolve. (Peter Marin, 1981)

In narrative practice, the emphasis is on the lived experiences of the person, not on interpretations of behaviors or the unconscious. Narrative practice makes use of this understanding of peoples' need to find new meaning in their lives, and it is this important element which serves as a motivator in narrative's emphasis on helping people to re-author their lives toward preferred outcomes. The re-authoring comes out of the social context of the person's lived experiences or to what White has often referred to as the total landscape of the person's life. What experiences in their past might be used to rekindle hope for the future? What had they wanted to be as they grew up? Had they ever had a job they enjoyed? Had they ever written for the school newspaper? Had they been active in civil rights, volunteered, and so forth?

WHO GOES THERE? STRANGER OR FRIEND?

The basic initial concern for the worker, knowing some of the feelings that exist in any new experience, is how to make this opening period of time comfortable for the client. Jay Haley (1971) suggests that the beginning of the first interview should emulate the welcome that you would give a guest coming to your home. While the physical setting may be out of your control, your welcome to the client is not. Like it or not the start of the session is usually under your control. Greetings are in order, protocols according to age and sex are in order, respect is in order, and patience is in order. The narrativists see the helping sessions as conversations rather than interviews, but conversations with a purpose. The purpose is to help the client work on what they want to see happen to them. You introduce yourself with a few words that are appropriate for the clients before you. They in turn are asked to do the same. The conversation may then turn to more specific items.

What is it they expect? What is the story that brought them here? How do they interpret the reasons they have come? Does everyone present see it the same way? What is the precipitating factor that has led to the visit? Have you given everyone an opportunity to present their view of what the situation may be?

While the worker is aware of these motivating factors in general, the circumstances for this particular individual are related to the way this person interprets the problem. We "know nothing" about the meaning of this experience to these participants or how reflective their narrative is of their actual experience.

Narrative Therapy does not begin with the problem; it begins with a conversation with the person coming to the worker about the things that brought him or her to you. The person is asked to tell their story in their own ways. The only questioning might be for clarity if things do not appear to be clear to the worker. If the worker is dealing with a family or group, then each member tells his/her version of the story. Later, as the person is more relaxed and past the initial anxiety of the meeting, the worker begins to ask the type of questions which begin to identify the nature of the problem. When appropriate, the problem is externalized, and may be given a name. White's questions "are rhetorical, designed to help people realize that: (1) they are separate from the problems, (2) they have power over the problems, and (3) they are not who they thought they were" (Nichols & Schwartz, 1998, p. 465).

DECONSTRUCTING THE STORY

One of the first tasks of the worker, requirement if you will, is dedicated listening. Not only listening for what is said, but also for what is missing from the story. Active listening is also an important indicator to the client that you care about what is being said. An important part of the listening process is assuming a "know nothing" frame of reference. That is, the worker asks the types of questions that arise out of the narrative, asking the client to fill in the gaps. The worker avoids making public assumptions about what might exist in those gaps, but realizes they may be crucial to the re-authoring process. Expanding on understanding what was unsaid, even though you as a worker may have heard similar stories before. You "know nothing" about the meaning of this story to this client.

The following is an excerpt from a social work student's meeting with a teenage girl sent by her school for counseling.

> During the first part of the conversation, Z and I were talking about what women should look like, and where people get the idea that "ultra" thin is the only figure women should have in order to be considered pretty.
>
> Z: Well, the movies, TV, magazines.
> W: It's hard not to start to think that's the way to look, has it influenced you?
> Z: I guess so, but I'm not really worried about food I eat O.K.
> W: Glad to hear that, sounds good. Are there times that you were worried about food?
>
> We talked a little about her eating, the diets she had been on, and supported her knowing she has to eat well and that she seemed to have come to terms with dieting, when she asked,
>
> Z: Do you know any exercises to help your waist get smaller?
> W: That's an interesting question, I guess we could find some, why do you want them?
>   Silence.
> W: Has weight been a problem for you?
>   Silence. Z, looking away.
> W: Do you think you are too heavy?
> Z: One of the guys I like, likes girls who are very thin, one day when we were at the mall, he looked at the manikins, and said he liked girls who looked like that.
>   She looked at me and laughed.

While workers know that teenage girls in general want to look thin and may start to starve themselves, the worker didn't know what was motivating this teenager. If the worker had just talked about exercise, part of the story would have remained lost. By trying to find out the "untold" the reasons become clear. Now there is room to start a re-authoring process, to discuss expectations and where the ideas about weight come from.

EXTERNALIZING THE PROBLEM

The externalizing of the problem, that is placing the problem in context outside of the person, suggests that the problem is not in the person and may have a life of its own independent of the person, the proof of which might be that many others also are battling the same problem. If people come for help believing themselves to be a problem or believing that their lives are just a series of problems, then both the client and the worker can be overwhelmed by an impossible task of dealing with a problem-saturated person or group. From the outset, efforts are made to separate the person from the problem. The person is asked a series of questions that inquire how the problem affects them. How does "guilt" get you to do things you would rather not do? How has "anger" led you to be placed in the detention home? How does "car-fear" keep you from having the kind of enjoyment in life you would like to have? White has a number of questions aimed at helping this externalizing process.

Nichols and Schwartz (1998) point out that, "Whether it's an internal experience (guilt, self-hate), a syndrome (anorexia, schizophrenia), or a relationship pattern (a rift), the externalized problem is always personified—portrayed as an unwelcome invader that tries to dominate the family members' lives" (p. 411).

Internalizing of the problem makes the person an object, rather than making the problem the object. How does internalizing the problem manifest itself? At the first session of the new semester, as students introduce themselves to the teacher and to each other, one or two will state their name and then add "and I am an alcoholic." This is an approach that they have been recruited into. It assumes that being able to admit to your problem is an important step in the recovery process. Indeed, it may be helpful to recognize that alcohol plays an important part in their lives. But is it an advantage to label yourself, and believe that you must live with that label all your life? They not only see themselves as a problem but they also take the problem into the class with them.

Narrative practitioners would not suggest that the person does not have a problem with alcohol, but would help the client see alcohol as the problem, and not themselves. They would seek ways to help persons understand the impact that alcohol has on their lives, and map the impact it has on others they are connected to as well. The mapping of the problem, which we discussed earlier, also permits discussion of who might be called upon as supports of the change process. Through a series of externalizing questions, the person is helped to recognize that while there are factors within them that may determine the nature of how they deal with the problem, these factors are not hidden and can be revealed, and are often related to something "out there" that needs to be dealt with, that can be resisted, controlled, and overcome. The problem is not within them, but they have been recruited to ways of thinking that place problems within the person. Clients are told that the work of both the client and the workers, and others when appropriate, will be directed at finding ways to overcome that problem.

Externalizing the problem tends to take the feeling of shame, guilt, and often hopelessness, off of the person. They are not bad because they drink, although the alcohol may cause them to behave in a manner which is hurtful to others and to themselves and can not be tolerated if others are hurt. Being an alcoholic is not something to be ashamed of, or to be branded with for life. Alcohol can be overcome if the person is willing to work on ways in which "Al" has started to control their lives. Not to see "Al" as an ally to be turned to when things go wrong, like a good friend; he is a bad friend, who will get you in trouble, and in reality is no friend at all, but an enemy to be resisted, fought, and subdued.

The nature of the questions which can help accomplish this renaissance of behavior are questions which relate the person's real life experiences to external problems. How does "Al" get you in trouble? What are some of the techniques "Al" has that get you to take a drink when you really don't want to? How has "Al" shown that he cares about you? Has "he" shown that he can hurt you rather then help? Under what circumstances does "Al" seem to have the most influence over you? When did "Al" recruit you into joining up with him? What was going on in your life at that time? Did "Al" have any influence on any of your family members when you were growing up? How does "he" impact them now?

Similar questions can be asked about any problem identified by the client as the cause of the current situation. It can be the hitter, or anger, or lazy-bone, and so forth. These questions permit the worker to gain an understanding of the impact of the problem, and at the same time, the client begins to gain a better understanding of his/her relationship to the problem. Some of the historical factors will emerge as the worker questions the person about "anger's" earlier involvement in his/her life, without asking the linear type question of whom else in your family is the angry one. That type of question places the "blame" in the family. In addition, it might serve to worry the client as to the biological/inheritable aspects of alcoholism, or anger, once again placing the problem within the person, rather than serving to externalize the problem.

Many of White's clients were women who came with stories of oppression by others, most often men, but possibly at times others. What he came to observe was that women are recruited by society to believe themselves to be unworthy or to be worthy only if they do what their husbands tell them, or are superb mothers, or are thin, or this, or that.

Questions seeking the source of these ideas of obedience, perfection, or humility would arise from the client's stories of trying to please others, often having a self-imposed obligation to do for others, while neglecting themselves. Or they feel shame for not living up to the expectations which they came to believe were the models of women in the social context and/or culture.

These beliefs become major forces in directing the person's life. The mutual task of worker and client as the helping process proceeds is to recognize where these external mandates are coming from, and how they serve the purposes of a select few, hardly ever the person seeking help, and how these forces which were external to the person have come to make the person believe they were the problem.

The person might then be asked, for example, how perfection has directed her life. How does perfection keep you from doing the things that you would like to be doing, from developing a new career, from maintaining a certain respect in the family, or to be treated differently by a spouse? Thus, a person learns that a male-oriented culture might have led her to believe that the only way to be accepted is to be the perfect wife or mother and that the pressure to be perfect forced her into devoting her life to the needs of others to the neglect of her own desires.

At times, this desire to be seen as perfect or acceptable has caused serious physical as well as emotional problems. This has proven to be particularly true with teenage girls and the overbearing pressure to be seen as having the right body. Achieving the perfect body often means not eating, eating a minimally nutritionally required diet, taking diet pills, or neglecting other life activities in order to lose weight. Anorexia has become a universal problem particularly for teenage girls but has become a major danger for adult women as well.

While it may be more difficult to help a teenager understand that there can be a life that differs from the norms set by her peers, the effort to externalize the problem of perfection or anorexia of the food monster, needs to be undertaken. Questions related to how anorexia became an expert on what she should eat, or where "it" got a degree in nutrition, while sounding frivolous or lighthearted, catches the attention of the teen who has seen numerous medical and mental health workers as her parents tried to help their ill child.

It sounds weird to start talking about something that wants to kill you, or somehow knows what you should be eating, and to talk about how this "thing" has started to take over control of your life. It may seem odd as well for a woman to talk about how "perfection" has led her to believe she is not a good wife or mother, how it tricks her into spending long hours in the kitchen when she might be doing something more appealing or something she never thought it was alright for women to do, such as seeking an advanced education. Yet, these are legitimate questions to ask, when there is an understanding and belief that certain social forces are at work leading that person to desperation and the healthy desire to want to change their life circumstances.

In White's seminal article on the externalization of the problem, he uses the case of a young child who soils. The externalization of the problem leads to the culprit as being "sneaky poo," so named because of both the relevance of the title and the idea that "poo" is tricky, someone to be watched and someone out there who is plotting at all times to get the child in trouble. For a child who was always being scolded for something, which for him was partially seen as fun, a plaything, the aim is to start to instill the idea that indeed "sneaky poo" was not his friend, not a playmate, and indeed was always getting him into trouble, particularly with his parents, but was also keeping him from enjoying certain other aspects of his childhood. For example, did he have any friends? He did not because of the displeasure being near him evoked.

It is with the externalizing process, that White's influence by people like Foucault becomes most clearly illustrated. While the childish activities rarely call for discussion of the major societal forces which shape a client's behavior, the work with adults, particularly women and minorities, illustrates the importance of externalization. Time and time again researchers have demonstrated how language and values held by socially upper class people are used to control, shape, and at times manipulate people along gender and ethnic lines (Illich, 1975).

The denial of opportunities for women is legend. Equal pay and educational opportunities are still marginally accepted in most countries. Discrimination against minorities, gays, and lesbians is still a major issue confronting the people in the United States with certain groups proclaimed as damned. Terms such as the unworthy poor and welfare cheats are still terms which tend to leave lasting scars on their recipients. There is a marginalizing process which generally relegates certain groups to the status of being inferior, less worthy, and at times a detriment to our society.

Racism and classism are very much alive and create systems of belief that are not only promulgated by the power structures, but also often accepted by those groups who are its targets. This is even more likely to be true when the language and tools of change are in the hands of those who will benefit by the oppressive labeling. It is this type of thinking which has led White and others to maintain that therapy too is a part of society and as a part of the powerful elements of society is often party to this oppressive practice. White would have us understand that therapy is a political process which is often used for the benefits of those in power. These beliefs echo the works of Foucault (1965, 1978) and Ivan Illich whose work on language and its control by the power structure demonstrates the politicization of the helping profession.

The growth of the DSM *(Diagnostic and Statistical Manual)* and its use as a mechanism of control, indeed for shaping those who can be seen as deviant, supports these views. Externalization of the problem avoids such labeling. There is no DSM number for "sneaky poo" or "loneliness" or "perfection." But it is possible to subvert those externalized problems into a scientific base that would meet the requirements of the DSM. Psychiatric diagnosis evolved from just two diagnostic categories, sane and insane, into the more than 100 different labels that are now listed. At one point homosexuality was included, and while now eliminated, there is still strong concern and dialogue around the actual existence of it as an "illness." In the tradition of deconstruction, one needs to ask, "who benefits by including such a category in the DSM?" Or better yet, who benefits from the DSM? Surely, for some people it is helpful to understand that there is a scientific term for something that "ails" them. There is some comfort in believing that what you have actually exists and can be named, and therefore can be dealt with. It is certainly of value to those who must share information about a client. It enables a common language and perhaps understanding. The validity, however, of the assessments is often brought into doubt when researchers attempt to gather proof that various therapists would agree on a diagnosis (Nylund, 1994; Tomm, 1998).

Labeling the problem may offer some sense of security, but as long as it remains internalized, the person feels the guilt, the shame, and the oppressiveness of the problem. In situations in which such a label is necessary, such as in the matter of insurance payment requirements, or agency regulations, some understanding can be reached with the client which explains the worker's requirements to attach the label, while pointing out that this is a political requirement, and that their own relationship to the problem may be seen quite differently.

For example, recently the discussion of whether "bigotry" should be labeled as a mental illness has been given a great deal of consideration. So has a suggestion that road rage be added as a DSM classification. The disputes as to what makes up mental illness, something that needs psychiatric care, are not new. Emily Eakin (2000) in a *New York Times* article writes:

> In 1851, Dr. Samuel A. Cartwright, a Louisiana surgeon and psychologist, filed a report in a New Orleans Medical and Surgical Journal on diseases prevalent among the South's black population. Among the various maladies Dr. Cartwright describes was "drapetomania" or the disease causing slaves to run away. Though a serious mental illness, drapetomania, wrote Dr. Cartwright, was happily quite treatable: "The cause, in most of the cases, that induces the Negro to run away from service, is as much a disease of the mind as any other species of mental alienation, and much more curable. With the advantage of proper medical advice, strictly followed, this troublesome practice that many negroes have of running away can be almost entirely prevented." (Eakin, p. A21)

If there is an inclination to think, "well that was then, and now we know better," think again. In a review of what the authors see as new developments to therapy, Gottlieb notes:

> Clinically inclined therapists have never had a problem with psychiatry's Diagnostic and Statistical Manual of Mental Disorders (DSM-IV), which ranges from the terrors of schizophrenia and manic depression to "Adjustment Reaction with Mixed Emotional Features" (that is being upset when something upsetting happens). (A. Gottlieb, 1997, p. 45)

One might wonder whether social workers upset about the mistreatment of a wife by her husband, a child by a parent, or even mistreatment of a client by the agency, would be reason to assign the worker DSM labels. The use of language to control is evidenced by categorizations like the DSM. While it may universalize workers' understanding of a problem, it also serves to endanger the future of persons in a society where the publicizing that a person has sought mental health help can ruin a career. This has happened a few times for those seeking political office and is extensive with those diagnosed as sex offenders.

THE RELATIONSHIP TO THE PROBLEM

In the course of the re-authoring process, some of the questions may relate to how the problem impacts the person in various situations; at home, on the job, or with friends. If it is a child, the parents might be expected to respond to how the problem impacts their lives as well. In this way, the parents of "sneaky poo" for example begin to see that they too must battle "poo." It is not a bad child that they must deal with but with the problem that is causing their child to behave in this undesired way. The mother did on occasion ignore the soiling, relaxed and took a break from letting "poo" control her life each day. The father was able to admit that poo kept him from talking about his child at work, like the other fathers were doing. This mapping process, exploring the extent that the problem impacts all the related persons, can lead to ways in which they start to change their thinking and their reactions to the problem. As the whole family begins to work at overcoming "poo" their relationship to him begins to change. They begin to feel more powerful and in control. They may work together thinking up strategies, and keep logs as to their successes.

Social workers have a good grasp of systems theory and how parts are in interaction and affect each other. This mapping process brings the parts into a living experience by exploring the actual impacts, how they operate, and how they change as the person begins to combat the problem. It moves away from the static view of a system and recognizes how forces external to the system can impact clients' lives. The maxim that no living system is a closed system becomes alive when an externalized problem starts to control some of the system's action.

The client can be helped to map their relationship to the problem. A simple scale of one to ten in which they show where they were when the work began, and where they are now, becomes an evaluative tool that can be very helpful in their understanding of how their relationship to the problem is changing. Tandy and Gallant (1993) present a more complex scale (see Figure 5.1).

UNIQUE EXPERIENCES

The continuing conversation often reveals times in which the problems may have been dealt with in unique ways—times in which the child did not "poo," times in which a client was able to ignore alcohol's call, when

A. To what extent has the problem of _____ been interfering with or dominating your life and relationships?
   (1) _____ rarely interferes with or dominates my life and relationships.
   (2)
   (3)
   (4)
   (5) Moderate interference
   (6)
   (7)
   (8)
   (9) _____ to an extreme extent has been interfering with or dominating my life and relationships.

B. Would you say the problem of _____ has been interfering with or dominating (what percentage) _____% of your life and relationships?

C. To what extent have you been successful in resisting the interference or domination of _____ in your life and relationships?
   (1) To no extent of success at all
   (2)
   (3)
   (4)
   (5) Moderate extent of success
   (6)
   (7)
   (8)
   (9) Successful resistance: _____ no longer dominates my life and relationships.

D. Would you say you have been (what percentage) _____% effective in resisting the interference or domination of _____?

[From Tandy, C., & Gallant, J. P. (1993). *Narrative therapy: A case study*. Unpublished manuscript, The University of Georgia, School of Social Work, Athens.]

FIGURE 5.1 Relative influence scale. This can be given a number of times over the course of helping. The same impact can be obtained by just drawing a line numbered 1 to 10 and asking the client to place him/herself on it related to the same type of questions above. It makes it less formal and test like. A variation might be to do it with other members of the family as well as the client.

agoraphobia was overcome in order to partake in some risky drive to an important family event. These incidents, no matter how trivial they may seem, provide evidence that the person is able to exert some control over the problem. If he/she can do it once, he/she can do it again.

The worker would spend careful time not only searching for the event, but also looking at where the person got the strength to do what was done. "What would your mom say if she knew what you were able to accomplish?" "Who else would be proud of what you have done?" "Who else shall we tell about your accomplishments?" If the worker is aware of other persons who were important in the client's life, the question of what that person would think about the accomplishment would be important as well. The family, of course, is one of the most vital shapers of the person's life, and family practice is on the cutting edge of the helping process.

FAMILY PRACTICE

Before there was family therapy, there was social work with families. In 1918, the *Annals* published an issue, *Social Work with Families*. It promoted "Social Case Treatment" with families including articles on working with The Normal Family, and The Fatherless Family. Even earlier, Mary Richman, a leader in the Charity Organization Society, wrote in her books about the social worker's relationship with the family. A book, *The Family and Social Work*, was written by Edward T. Devine in 1922 (Devine, 1922). He was the director of what is now the Columbia University School of Social Work. It is interesting that the earliest efforts in narrative practice were with families and that the family therapists picked it up more extensively than social work practitioners because early in its development social work was most prominent in working with families and in fact was one of the first professional groups to do so.

In the 1950s, social work started to work more therapeutically with the family as a family, recognizing the value of looking at the interactions among the family members, rather than looking at the individual in the family. Part of this was the growing recognition of the power of the group and the understanding of the social sciences. A major influence in the incorporation of social science knowledge into social work was Grace Longwell Coyle, whose seminal article looking at the family as a group was published in *Social Casework* in 1962. Coyle, a group work professor at Case Western Reserve School of Applied Social Sciences, noted that "for a long period of time the dynamic concepts of human behavior derived from psychiatry served to focus casework practice primarily on his (her) intra-psychic problems" (Coyle, 1958, p. 347). As the Freudian perspective began to lose its privileged place to other social science concepts, the dynamics of the environment and family life started the call for different practice approaches.

Most of the current writing relating to Narrative Therapy has appeared in the Family Therapy literature. It is appropriate, therefore, to search out some of the important elements that seem to make it so popular in that arena. We will not spend too much time trying to define what a family is. Hartman gives a definition we think worthy of adapting for our needs (Hartman & Laird, 1983).

> Such a family group in our context consists of two or more people who have made a commitment to share living space, have developed close emotional ties, and share a variety of family roles and functions. (p. 30)

(We view this as including single parent families).

Defining Family Therapy is another matter. While it would seem that it means working with the family as a unit, a great deal of the literature seems to be a practitioner with a single client. Perhaps the family might have been initially involved, but other family members appear rarely if at all in the subsequent meetings. Is this unique in Narrative Therapy? In their examination of research efficacy in family therapy, the editors of one journal (Goldstein, 1998) define family in a number of ways including: involving family members beyond the index person. This would suggest that at least two family-related participants need to be in direct communication with the worker in order to be considered Family Therapy. While on the surface this may seen a simple enough criteria, a closer look suggests some difficulties. Two come to mind. What should be the case if an HIV-infected person does not want anyone else to know of their situation? Should that person be discontinued as a client? What if a teenager seeking an abortion wants to discuss this with the therapist, but does not want her parents to know? Is this a proper case for Family Therapy as defined by the Journal's criteria? While these may seem exceptions, they raise ethical concerns, and certainly there are many other situations which would test the criteria, such as a divorce, or death of a spouse, or one partner deciding not to go for help after an initial meeting or two. Exceptions aside, there certainly are benefits to working with the family as an entity, as those familiar with systems theory will attest, and most family therapists would see family practice as the major foundation of their work.

Salvador Minuchin, for one, seems to believe so, and raises the question, "Where is the family in Narrative Therapy?" (Minuchin, 1998). Having observed some narrative therapists at a workshop, Minuchin (1999) believes they are ignoring the family, and only dealing with individuals. Part of Minuchin's reactions may be due to his general questioning of the efficacy of deconstructive approaches. Earlier writings reflect some of his concerns (Minuchin, 1991).

Michael White certainly works with the family and I doubt that he has ever suggested that Narrative Therapy was a helping model only for families, or not for families, and we would be surprised were he to do so. His work with sneaky poo certainly involved the family, and they were asked to look at the influence of sneaky poo on it. This view of the relationship to the problem was part of the mapping process, which he incorporates into his work. Later in his work with a group in a mental hospital, there is no indication that the family is involved, but he works with the hospitalized participants as a group and community. Narrative practice is not limited to work with families, and in fact it is its universal application to all sized social units that these authors see as a major breakthrough for a general practice model.

AN ORGANIZING PROCESS

Epston and Roth (1994) have presented an excellent framework for what they call the White/Epston type of interview. It offers the helper an organized way to begin the helping process. It includes:

Developing externalizing conversations; beginning by externalizing the problem.
Mapping the influence of the problem in the person's/family's life and relationships.
Mapping the influence of the person/family in the life of the problem.

Within this section of their framework they list and discuss a number of the types of questions they use in the helping process. Some of these are discussed below.

Unique account questions

Unique rediscription questions (These invite people to develop meaning from the unique accounts they have identified as they re-describe themselves, others, and their relationships.)

Unique possibility questions

Preference questions

Consulting your consulting questions (These serve to shift the status of a person from client to consultant.)

This latter series of questions amplifies the importance that Narrative Therapy places on the idea that the worker not be seen as the expert. The idea is that the client is his/her own best consultant. Other processes such as the reflecting team supports those efforts. It is important to note as well that a great deal of the helping that takes place is due to the style of questioning, and to the belief that the questions lead to reflection by the client, and are in the service of the client, rather than the helper.

We see an additional factor as extremely important in this helping process and one which is particularly reflected in the narrative approach, and that is *listening*. We have noted the vital part that worker client relationship plays in the success of the helping particularly from the viewpoint of the client. The belief by the client that the worker really is listening to his/her story, and attentive to the importance it has in his/her life is crucial in the helping process. Listening, no matter how trivial or irrelevant the context may seem, has an important impact on the client. The ability to see that the worker is listening transforms the talk to a thoughtful narrative.

6

The Written Word:
Letters and Logs and Briefs

Writing was also important in the culture of taking care of oneself. One of the main features of taking care involved taking notes on one to be reread, writing treatises and letters to friends to help them, and keeping notebooks in order to reactivate for oneself the truths one needed.

Foucault

If you don't write it down it never happened.

(Comment to social work students)

The use of case materials is a mainstay of the social work profession (Lawson & Prevatt, 1999). Everyone in social work and similar helping disciplines is familiar with the use of records and their stated importance. Those who have worked in the public welfare services are only too familiar with the stacks of written materials that accompany each case and are mandated in the name of accountability. Historically, in the Charity Society days, the first recordings were to document the distribution of resources and were nothing more than a ledger. They contained the type of material that currently would appear on the face sheet of current case records.

As the profession evolved, it became more important to indicate why the resources were being distributed to particular parties and what effect it had. These recordings included ". . . . detailed reports of day-to-day contacts with clients as well as judgements regarding clients' needs and the consequences of the help. Thus, the narrative record came into being" (Kagle, 1987, p. 463). These soon evolved into process recordings which offered more of a verbatim record of what both the worker and the client said. This served as a means of enhancing understanding of the helping process, and to further sociological interpretations that could be used for research purposes.

While clinical records are generally a requirement in most agencies, for both legal and funding reasons, their original use was as a narrative case recording describing the helping process. They became a major teaching and learning tool that remains in use to this day. With the large caseloads that many workers in child welfare have, they also serve as a reminder for the busy worker of where the process had left off at the last meeting. The vast amount of required forms has created situations in which few workers have the time to do process recordings in some settings.

For those working on developing their approach or developing a new approach, the recordings become a search for material that support their views by illustrating concrete examples of the points they were trying to make. Further, it offered the opportunity to codify something that had been a transient verbal interactive process into a document which had body and substance, and which could be reviewed and used. One of the major purposes of writing records is to reflect on them after the meeting and to think about how you would have approached that situation the next time. Would you have done it the same way? If things didn't go "right," looking at the recording may give you some clues as to what might have gone wrong. At what point did this begin to move in a direction that deterred the process from being helpful?

While the course of a session could be reconstructed at a later time, the reconstruction was often subject to distortions, additions, or omissions because of the contingencies of the person's memory, to the purpose for which the recording was going to be used. If it wasn't written down, it never happened. This was a particularly salient point when the supervisory conference came around. The supervisee's responses as to what "really" happened could be constructed and reconstructed on the spot. There was no grounded recording that could be used as a basis for the examination of what really happened with the client.

Holland (1991) in discussing the values of narrative writes,

> The development and analysis of the case history is a powerful but underutilized tool for guiding social work practice. Rather than a mere record or chronicle of events, the client's story is the doorway to understanding how meaning has struggled to emerge in this life. Effective participation in the process of finding and developing meaning can be enhanced by means of a broad acquaintance with other life stories . . . (Holland, 1991, p. 39)

In this 1991 article, Holland does not yet appear to be familiar with the Narrative Therapy literature, as none appears in his bibliography. He does, however, point out the value of narrative for the practitioner, particularly as a way of understanding.

While any recording is subject to the maxim "everything written is written by an observer," it might be fair to say that if the situation is not written down, it never happened. It is lost. It is only in the memory, subject to forgetting, adlibbing, or may vanish completely if the therapist never records it. This is a particularly important point in the larger agency where many workers may be involved with a client or family over an extended period of time. There have been examples of lost or misplaced cases and of resulting damage including deaths because no one was keeping up with the case, particularly in child abuse situations.

Case materials, summaries, and records of accountability have been historically demanded of the therapist. They add to the permanency of a situation. They permit reflection and comparison. Their initial use was for accountability and growth for oneself. With the evolution of case management, recordkeeping has become a required task of the worker if they are to be reimbursed for their services, and in conjunction with the DSM has become a mainstay of clinical practice. Therapists introducing new approaches to helping often depend on their case material to serve as a substitute for evidence of effectiveness, since with a small sample the ability to do quantitative research is limited. Generally these records have always been seen as confidential. Although this has been seen as a means of ensuring client confidentiality, the records are rarely shared with the clients. While it is reasonable to establish the utmost security in maintaining the records safely from the eyes of the wrong people, it is not as clear as to the reasons to keep the records from the eyes of the client. Overall confidentiality is of vital importance when the revelation of the contents could be used against a person, for political reasons or economic/job possibilities. This is particularly true of the material furnished to welfare departments where the provision of public funds often carries a threat of the political misuse of recipients' names.

Bacigalupe (1996) points out, as does White, that the therapeutic encounter occurs in the context of wider social relationships. This includes the writing of case material.

> Therapy may re-create the same social relationships that exist "outside" of the clinical context. Although as therapists we may strive to be "neutral," we bring our particular values and location in society into the session. What we discuss and write about with clients is influenced by age, gender, race, and social class and our position of often being outsiders to the world

of clients. In this regard, postmodern systemic therapists, have recognized the encounter of therapists and clients as being like that of the native and the ethnographer in anthropological fieldwork. (p. 362)

Writing with individuals, groups, and family therapy has been used to help clients in a number of ways. Behavior therapists will often ask clients to record their or their children's activities as a means of establishing boundary lines and assessing change. Ira Progoff's (1975) work on intensive journals, which he started to develop in 1965, was used as a therapeutic writing device in order to aid the client in self-evaluation and forward projection. Progoff writes,

> The Intensive Journal plays an active role in reconstructing a life, but it does so without imposing any external categories or interpretations or theories on the individual's experience. It remains neutral and open-ended so as to maintain the integrity of each person's development, while drawing him further along the road of his (her) own life process. . . . The Intensive Journal is specifically designed to provide an instrument and techniques by which persons can discover within themselves the resources they did not know they possessed. (Progoff, 1975, pp. 9–10)

The reader might note above some verisimilitude with the ideas of narrative practice, the avoidance of giving too much direction, the stress on the autonomy of the client, and the process of reconstructing a life. Clients have been asked to write autobiographies, or stories, of their lives. Some clients have expressed themselves in poems, and numerous clients have written about their therapeutic experience, both the successes and failures, and some have become best sellers (Martin, 1992).

Freud has been known to have written to clients and used the letters themselves in a therapeutic manner. He was gracious about responding, often responding to strangers who would ask for his help. All of his responses, even to strangers, were cordial and attempted to be helpful given the limitations of the brief encounters. In one situation he interpreted a women's dreams in a manner which might give her some clues to her life situation, even though he notes he can do very little without further information from her. This correspondence and Freud's use of letter writing is discussed in Ludy and Diyon (1966).

Bacigalupe, recognizing the importance of the written correspondence between the therapist and the client, makes it a point to recommend increasing that type of communication (Bacigalupe, 1996, p. 361). He fosters efforts to use this mutual writing as a means of therapy, suggesting that it encourages therapeutic participation. His review of a number of efforts in which this mutual writing has proven to be valuable suggests it can add to the collaborative efforts between therapist and client. He also suggests there is value in the clients writing autobiographies.

LETTERS

In discussing the difference between the narrative mode of thought from the logic-scientific, Epston and White (1990) say that the narrative mode is characterized by good stories that gain credence through life experience. The lived experience is privileged over reified constructs and categories. Time becomes important because stories are related to plots that unfold over time. Of course language is extremely important in narrative, not only as a form of expression between the worker and the client, but because of the way it was used in society for power and subjugation. We see the use of written language as useful in the practice of letter writing that Epston and White utilize to help clients.

They have listed a series of types of letter, which we will mention briefly:

1. Letters of invitation. These serve to engage people in therapy who are reluctant to attend.
2. Redundancy Letters. Letters that make people redundant in such roles as "parent watcher" or "brother's father." A particularly moving one is a letter written by a mother to her twelve-year-old son who has been taking care of her for many years. It starts, "Dear Danny, I am writing you this letter thanking you for your services over the past eight years of your life" (p. 91).
3. Letters of prediction. These are usually done at the end of therapy, and project a future of about 6 months. They can serve as a review for the client, but might also act as a prophecy that can fulfill itself.
4. Counter-referral letters. Letters back to a referral source, pointing out the positives that have taken place and the strengths of the person.
5. Letters of Reference. Letters that can be used to show people that the person has made changes, and is competent.
6. Letters for special occasions. Examples are a letter related to the feelings a person has had about a memorial service for his brothers and the guilt involved. Another to people who were pressuring a young girl who had been raped. It explains her behavior in relation

to the trauma involved, and suggests, "If you want to help Julie, give her time and space to heal and recover her mind from terror and the nightmare she lived through" (p.107).

There are short letters written to clients following a meeting. These are often a review and help carry over the important processes of the meeting. They aid in the continued re-authoring processes, raising things to think about, providing support, and helping the person act as an observer of the change that has been taking place.

None of the modern therapies, however, have made use of writing as a therapeutic tool in the way that White and Epston have been able to do. One chapter of their book is devoted to letter writing which they have categorized into various letter types such as letters for special occasions, counter-referral letters, and brief letters. Within these groups are sub-headings, Therapist Needs Help, and Challenging the Techniques of Power. These letters are often used in place of case notes. Epston has noted that these often serve as the only record he might have of a meeting with a client. While this may seem odd to many of us used to having to furnish record material and assessments to insurance companies, this may not be a problem in New Zealand where a form of socialized medicine might provide a less demanding reporting ritual. Many of my students were told by their agencies that they should not write letters to clients when I asked them to check out whether or not this would be allowed under agency policy. In most cases the reason was given that it was against agency policy, although no evidence of such written policies were available.

The first time I taught my Narrative Therapy course a student wrote a letter to a client. His supervisor was not familiar with this approach and called the school to find out more about it. The agency-faculty contact also was unaware of letter writing and an education process ensued. After a number of years teaching the course, many of the agencies are aware of its uses and some have permitted the students to write letters to the clients after reviewing them with the supervisor.

Epston suggests that at times letters are specifically written to be shared with others and this is mentioned to the client, while some are labeled confidential (White & Epston, 1990). In an article in the *Family Networker* edited by O'Hanlon (1994), Epston discusses the use of letters, their importance, and the research that has been done to assess their effectiveness. In some of his workshops he has elaborated on the importance of letter writing (Epston, 1996). What does letter writing accomplish?

There is something about seeing things in writing that makes it more believable than being told about it. We are more likely to accept the truth of the written word. In addition, we can re-read it, and confirm the words, and while we can interpret that statement in different ways, we cannot change the actual words. Being told that you are making progress in therapy or that you were not to blame, but have been misused, has a different impact when told to you by the therapist versus getting a letter in the mail saying the same thing. So on the face of it, having something in hand, something solid, a letter, adds an important element to the helping session.

In addition, it serves not only as a continuation of the process that took place in the last session, but also can be a connection to the next session while enabling work between the sessions. For example, in writing to the client about the change you believed has been taking place, you might ask her how she sees the process, or where she found the strength to challenge "big trouble." In an article "The Third Wave," Bill O'Hanlon also discusses the use of letter writing, and particularly a letter written to a woman who had told Epston at the first interview ". . . I'm bad! I'm bad! I'm bad." She had been abused all her life, physically and mentally. His lengthy letter to her outlined some of her life, and how she had been exploited and taught to see herself as bad. It also discussed the strengths she must have had in order to be able to have survived such oppressive treatment, and how she was gaining power from within herself. Several weeks later at another session with Epston, she told him how she had reread the letter many times. It was, she said, "reality" there in black and white, and she could not deny it. As a result she now saw herself as a person who had a terrible life but had always been strong and never submitted completely to a devalued view of herself (O'Hanlon, pp. 19–20).

While many of the letters are for the private viewing of the clients, there are times when the letter's purpose is to provide an audience or support group for the individual. For example, a child might have a letter indicating how his/her problem is being opposed and the changes that are taking place. This might be shown to the teacher as a way of helping s/he to understand the progress and what the child is working on. Another situation might be a letter to show to friends explaining why you appreciate their desire to help you at this time, but why you don't want to discuss things with them. Or even a letter that might say you have found your new self and that serves as an invitation to a gala "coming out" party.

Parry and Doan (1994) discuss some of the reasons that they use letters in their counseling. The first is to ensure that they have heard the client's story correctly, and the second is that it provides time for them to ponder the case outside of the therapeutic conversations. It extends the effect of therapy; it renders a new story more noteworthy through documentation; the client can compare the old story with the new; it expands the worker-client relationship (pp. 167–168).

We have found that when we asked our students to write letters to the client they were discussing in class, they reported that it made them feel closer to the client, and also that they were giving something to the client. It also opened up an important discussion about their concern as to whether or not they should be communicating with clients once the client is no longer being served by the agency. One student discussed an agency policy which suggested workers not send a Christmas card to a client, even if the client mails one to the worker. The subsequent discussion as to who might benefit from such a policy and who might suffer added an important dimension to their understanding of how rules are set, and how people are made to feel different from others in society by certain policies which suggest that they might in some way be "using" the Christmas cards in a manipulative, or nontherapeutic manner. Other students likewise had experiences in which they were told contact after a case was closed was not appropriate. The best reason the students were able to get from the agency was that that was the rule and there might be legal problems (not defined).

A number of students who would have liked to write letters to their clients were not permitted to do so. I suggested that they write the letters anyway, but not send them, just keep them, and we could discuss them, or if the opportunity arrived they might discuss them with the supervisor in the agency. Some of the students have mentioned how the writing itself made them consider their practice and the client in a different way, reflecting more carefully. They also noted how differently they would state things about the client, knowing that the client would be reading it. Most of those unspoken thoughts dealt with the strengths of the client. Is it possible that it is difficult to talk to clients about things they do well? Is it a concern that this might come across as false or as an attempt to "jolly" the client out of feeling poorly? It may be that the education that most helpers receive emphasizes a search for the problem, and positive conversation in which acknowledged accomplishments are noted has not received the emphasis that it should in the education of helpers. In addition the letter is future-oriented, helping the client think of what they might want to discuss at the next meeting. Similarly the letter as it is being written is a plan for the future by the worker.

As far as I know only two students shared their letters with the supervisor. In both cases the students had expressed being familiar with some of the ideas of Narrative Therapy prior to taking the course. This may be an indication of how difficult it is to actually incorporate new ideas into practice, particularly when there is little support for it in the agencies.

RE-LEARNING TO WRITE

While the title of this section might seem a little condescending, let me say that it is meant only to suggest that there are some techniques in writing therapeutically syntonic letters that can be helpful. Furthermore the authors recognize that we are not living in an age where people write letters. It is easier to call or to e-mail than to take the time to write a letter, stamp and address the envelope, and post it. Modernity and e-mail have enabled the shortened note and the brief conversation to replace reflective correspondence.

A student having trouble in school might be asked to write a letter to his teacher, explaining some of the problems he is working on, rather than the therapist doing it. They could talk together about what the child might want to say. A woman might be asked to write an autobiographical sketch based on the history she presented to the therapist. The client might be asked "If you were I (the worker) how would you write up today's meeting?" Each of these needs to be done in the context of the situation being worked on and the ability of the person to carry out the task. These collaborative efforts begin to place more of the power in the hands of the client as s/he begins to author his/her own material.

Bacigalupe (1996) has prepared a number of ways of engaging trainees as to the relationship of writing and therapy. He helps students address the oppressive dimensions that case documentation might hold for the lived experiences of worker and client. He asks, "How would your clinical practice change if you were not able to take notes during or after the therapy session?" and "If you were your client, would you like to be pictured in the text as you represented your client?" Attempting to alert the students to the impact of the institution on client and worker, he asks, "How much of your writing is done having in mind supervisors, colleges, clients, insurance companies . . ." (p. 371). Concluding, the author notes,

Hopefully, these ideas challenge the tendency to perceive therapists' mission as isolated from a commitment to social justice. The movement from writing about and to clients to writing with clients is a step forward in integrating collaborative, reflexive and liberating aspects of postmodern systemic therapy. (p. 372)

As part of the examination of letters written to clients it is interesting to discuss their power as seen by White and Epston. Their limited research with practitioners who have used letter writing indicates that these people believe a letter might be therapeutically equivalent to three sessions. Some helpers believe it to be equal to five visits. On the face of it this might seem grandiose, but we should not underestimate the power of the written word. Still it is important to consider that the responses are from people who are invested in the success of the narrative method. Further research on letter writing and on narrative's effectiveness in general is being carried out.

We believe that it is important to note the value of writing letters can have for the worker as well as the client. Writing stimulates the reflective, thoughtfulness of the communication. It helps the worker consider and revisit some of the ideas that he/she wants the client to hear that will help move the process forward. It can be such an anabling process that the writing of a letter by the client to the helper should also be considered as a valuable part of the work they do together. The client might be urged to do so if they believe it might be important for them to do so.

The use of poems and other "artistic" endeavors can also serve as examples of both client strength and creativity, and reflects parts of the landscape of their lives not available in other ways.

At times it is difficult to put into words some of what we have seen and heard. Weingarten (2000) notes in a version of a speech she presented in South Africa the words of Antjie Krog who covered The Truth and Reconciliation hearings. "Stunned by the knowledge of the price people have paid for their words. If I write this, I exploit and betray. If I don't, I die" (Krog, 1998, p. 66). Weingarten's article indicates some of the importance of narratives as "witness" and in helping understand cultural impact on community.

7

Groups and Communities

The Committee for the
Advancement of Social
Work with Groups

First Annual Symposium

SOCIAL WORK WITH GROUPS

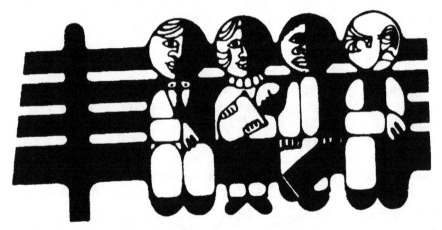

NOVEMBER 29, 30, DECEMBER 1, 1979

Hollenden House
Cleveland, Ohio

(The cover of the first symposium on Social Work With Groups. The mural
"Life is Sharing the Same Park Bench" by the artist John Morrell of
Rochester NY, is in Cleveland, Ohio. It has become the logo of the
Association for the Advancement of Social Work with Groups which formed
following this symposium. The authors were the symposium coordinators)

"The Low Road" (Excerpt)

What can they do
to you? Whatever they want . . .

It goes on one at a time,
it starts when you care
to act, it starts when you do
it again after they said no,
it starts when you say We
and know who you mean, and each
day you mean one more.

(*The Moon is Always Female.* Marge Piercy)

The small group acts as a mediator between the individual and the society. Persons learn through groups to accomplish certain life tasks and to work toward re-authoring their lives. Starting with their experiences as part of a family, it is the group that offers security and opportunity and shapes some of the thinking and doing of the individual. It is a tool for making connections with other persons and with institutions. Persons join with others for many reasons, including economic, educational, security, religious, and social-cultural-political reasons. The group becomes the means or tool that people can use on their own behalf and for others in mutual aid. The central concern around which persons organize becomes the "point of concentration" for the group's deliberations and actions. In the helping group, the point of concentration is the work that must be done to accomplish the desired future that the group members and the group find as a common ground around which to help each other with the added assistance of a worker.

White (1995a) recognizes the importance of the group and uses it in many ways. One of the most well known is the reflective team, which in itself is also an experience in mutual aid. This is discussed more fully in chapter 5. He also uses groups as an audience to the changes that are taking place in the lived experience of the individual and as a source of verifying the change. Another major use is as a support group. White suggests its use as a counterforce to the abuse team and calls it the "nurturing team." He and the client extend invitations to join the nurturing team: "If there is a shortfall in membership, therapists can put people in touch with others who are 'card carrying' nurturing team members who would be willing to play the part" (White, 1995a, p. 105).

The small group is a response and a counterforce to increased deper-sonalization, accelerated mechanization, and blatantly indifferent institu-tions. There is a growing recognition that groups provide a vital context, not only for individual growth and social change, but also for enriched relationships among people and between people and their institutions. Recent societal trends have started to destroy many of the personal bonds and connections or what Putnam (2000) calls "social capital" (*Bowling Alone*). The importance of the group in people's lives has particular sig-nificance for the field of social work and in narrative practice. When the small group mobilizes and starts to make connections with other groups, the social action or community organization aspect of the social work field is brought into focus.

In this section we will examine some of the efforts of practitioners to use narrative with groups. Organizing groups for social action provides a means to counter some of the power that some persons and organizations have over the lives of others. Many oppressed groups, welfare mothers, prisoners, and minorities of many kinds have been able to wrest some power into their own hands through organization. Narrative's focus on contextual issues is a natural part of the approach. It deals with the reality that the social context may be involved in how the person perceives their relationship with the problems. In social work, it is not an added-on effort for the worker to do social action. It is part of the expectations, noted as a mandate in the code of ethics. Social action is what the worker does, and change, both individual and social, involves working together with others. There can be individual change in the person's feelings about themselves or in their landscape of consciousness, but it can only be demonstrated and tested out in behaviors, usually with others.

People learn through groups to accomplish certain life tasks and to work for desired ends. Not only does the group shape the person's life, but it also becomes a tool which the person can use on his/her own behalf or on behalf of others. During the past thirty to forty years, the group has become a major tool in the mental health field and is increas-ingly seen as effective in therapy. In social work, the small group covers a great deal of territory. The first uses of groups in social work were related to the settlement movement (Coyle, 1958; Lubove, 1965; Woods, 1970) and has come to be referred to as the social goals model, since a great deal of the work of the settlement was aimed at helping people, particularly newly arrived persons, to become good citizens and learn the American way of life. Small group work moved into the therapeutic arena shortly after World War I, working with the Red Cross and the returning veterans

(Walkowitz, 1999). The model most prevalent at this point is more general and is generally referred to as the interactional model. Formulated by William Schwartz, it takes a more generalist systems model that suggests that group work can carry multi-functions, including social goals, treatment, social action, and prevention. It has also been known as the mediating model, since Schwartz held that the function of the worker with the group was to mediate the process by which the individual and the group reach out for each other in mutual aid (Pappell & Rothman, 1966; Schwartz, 1961).

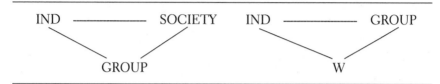

Interactional patterns of social group work

There is a range of uses of the group in social work. These include socialization groups for children and adults, therapeutic groups and support groups, reminiscing groups for senior citizens, social action and community organizations encompassing political change groups that might want to change laws about bars in their community, and tenant groups in public housing (Abels, 1971, 1984; Gitterman & Shulman, 1994).

Dean (1998) itemizes a number of strategies for working with narratives in groups. The first deals with, *listening, validating, and bearing witness.* The telling and the responses from others can be very helpful and lead to new perspectives. *Exchanging and expanding stories* by the members involves interaction and building on each other's stories. It would seem that it would enhance communication and interaction among the members. Dean also suggests *reacting, questioning, and exploring.* Her brief discussion of *"externalizing problems and creating preferred accounts"* suggests that the worker ask the kinds of questions that would be asked in an individual session to externalize the problem. It seems the work here is done by the worker and no mention is made of the group doing the questioning. Changing "blaming" stories by challenging assumptions is another strategy that can be helpful in pointing out some of the patterns of the group's members and the way they approach the conversations in the session (Dean, pp. 31–35).

Dean has done a nice job in reviewing material on the narrative approach and how it might be used in groups. The use of the group members as helpers offers a major opportunity to increase the ability to help, by offering differing views and many "workers," but its use is often neglected. In social group work, the workers are committed to use the group as helpers, as context, and as an audience to their own change. This type of use of group is often missing in the group and family therapy oriented literature. It is often seen as feedback, which is valuable, but the idea of being an audience to your own change is not generally referred to outside of the narrative literature.

The essence of social group work, as in social work in general, is the process between persons, one of whom, the worker, carries the professional responsibility for promoting the process. It is within the process that individual and group change takes place and persons re-author their lives. The worker helps the group members utilize the group for change, and it is in the understanding of the importance of the process and its use that the skill of the worker manifests itself. The demand for work is a legitimate use of worker influence. Challenging what keeps the members from plotting some direction, questioning why they privilege one way of working, that is, autocratic, or bullying procedures, over another approach, is the way the group is helped to re-author the group story, and their own. While the worker has little contact with the lived experiences of the members outside the group, there is the hope that as they are able to re-author their lives in the group, they can use the same processes to re-author their lives outside the group. In a sense the group becomes the training ground for learning how to rewrite one's narrative. It is part of the person's story, though only a small part.

The group discussed in a previous chapter, in which the boys took on the roles of comic book heroes, was a group formed for a number of purposes. On one hand it became a "social club," which met the usual needs of the children to interact with others, and make friends. It was used by the mental health center for diagnostic purposes and by the parents as a way to have their children have a good time.

Irving Yalom (1995), a psychiatrist who was instrumental in getting traditional psychotherapists interested in the use of the group for therapeutic purposes, lists eleven therapeutic factors that he believes benefit the group members. While the list may not be exhaustive, it does illustrate what tools may be available to both members and workers in the re-authoring process. They include: Instillation of Hope, Universality, Imparting Information, Altruism, The Corrective Recapitulation of the Primary Family Group, Development of Socializing Techniques, Imitative Behavior, Catharsis, Existential Factors, and Group Cohesiveness (Yalom, 1995).

While we have discussed constructivism earlier and its belief that knowledge is historically and culturally bound, it is relative in working with groups to recall that knowledge, according to Bruner (1990), is a by-product of the stories transmitted by that culture's psychology and use of language. "Implicit in such a belief system is the idea that culture is not an objective entity but, rather a social creation or invention. Constructivism, therefore, emphasizes the importance of the social context in the formation of individual meaning" (Levine, 1997, p. 197). The social context is exactly what the small group provides. It becomes a cultural milieu in which the member interacts with others, both shaping and being shaped by the nature of the communication that takes place. When the worker is able to make use of the members as helpers, this "culture" is a formative factor in helping the members re-author their lives. The group becomes both audience and co-authors in the process.

In prison, opportunities to experience real life problems, to find extensive support, and to change behaviors are limited. However, time and talk are plentiful. Sheridan (1995) notes the importance of stories and spirituality in work in prisons with groups (1995, p. 3):

> "I like that saying, 'Real Talk,'" said Mark. "It's different from the talk in here [the general prison] population." I asked him to be specific. Keven volunteered, "Here the talk is quieter, and there's less bullshit. People are trying to learn something. It's real. It makes you feel like you've got a brain and a life." Mark said, "Right. Out there, war stories about drugs and broads are like drugs. You turn off feelings. You're cool. You don't have to think." (Albert, pp. 210–211)

At the next meeting the members are talking about sex and how they have lost the power that they used to have.

> After a silence, Mark said very slowly and soberly, "you're in the limelight when you got the product [cocaine]. Everyone comes to you: women, friends. I feel like I'm giving up everything. I'm afraid recovery will be lonely." I let this sink in. Then I asked if others were afraid of being lonely. Almost everyone was. With each admission, it was as if shadows were lifted. Finally, the discussion turned to strategies other than sex and drugs for avoiding loneliness. (p. 212)

The ability of the men to express that they too were concerned about loneliness helps clarify what type of work the men can help each other with in order to overcome the fear of loneliness which might hinder the ability to get out. They also shared ways they could overcome loneliness.

While this is very close to helping the group externalize the problem of "loneliness," some questioning about how to overcome loneliness rather than avoid it makes for a more active role in providing the client with a sense of urgency. Subsequent conversations might look at the "unique experiences," times when the person overcame loneliness without drugs, and how loneliness recruited him/her into using drugs. A final comment on this—in a group situation the other members are also helpers and can be involved in sharing their experiences in resisting loneliness and its demands on them. In some situations discussion with the members of any group, particularly members living in a "total institution," about how the institution might help, or what hinders the change, can lead to another form of action of benefit not only to themselves, but also to helping the institution in achieving its goals.

We are reminded of the differences of work with Vietnam veterans in which some therapists saw the veterans as emotionally ill, and psychopathological, and assigned them diagnostic labels such as "Neurotic Guilt" (Haley,1974). Others saw the "treatment" as recognizing that the veterans themselves were victims and involved the veterans in "rap" groups to talk about what happened to them and what they might do about it. This led to actions to protest the war and to become active in other aspects of social change. It also led to a self-help movement of veterans around mental health issues. This was a way of giving the participants a sense of control over their lives and helping them deal with the pain of what they had done (Haley, 1974; Shatan, 1973).

Levine (1997) presents a case with an individual who had been diagnosed as Attention Disorder ADHD. As the presentation unfolds, we see how all of the groups with which the client has had contact over the years from schoolroom to teachers and even the family are impacted by the diagnosis he was given as a child. "The broad research concerning the ramifications of bearing a psychiatric diagnosis reveals that, in general, individuals so identified are shunned by others" (Link & Sullivan, 1998, p. 202).

Aaron Brower (1996) writes that constructivism focuses on how people create meaning in the lives, and "nowhere is this more clearly seen than in group work, a modality that forces members to develop a shared understanding of the treatment setting" (Brower, 1996, p. 336). He believes that the group must be brought along from collections of individuals to a coordinated group with shared perceptions and meanings. He goes on to create a "constructivist model of group development." The first stage is anomie or normlessness, citing Yalom's idea that when we cannot make sense of a situation, anomie confronts us head-on with the anxiety of being "at-sea" or "groundless." Yalom sees himself as an existentialist therapist (Yalom, 1980.) Group members then develop a "schema" of personal rules. We might see this as a personal story of how one is to act in certain situations. Because they have to interact with each other in the group, and they are strangers to each other, they often violate each other's schemas, leading to increased confusion. The leader (worker) explains the rules which become the reality for the group. "To the extent that the leader (worker) provides an adequate vision for the members, the level of anxiety caused by anomie is reduced" (Brower, p. 338). The next phase is the members turning to each other, to seek a group vision they can live with rather than the worker's vision. This leads to the development of shared schemas.

Brower believes that a constructivist framework is very useful in helping clients make changes in their lives,

> . . . the language of constructivisim and schemas can create a mindset for clients that facilitates change. Constructivist tenets and language state that life is a creative and constructive process as opposed to a corrective process. Clients are therefore helped through constructive language to recognize that they are doing the best they can given what they know and perceive. At the same time, they are provided with the language to understand that the truth that they find in their lives is their truth and not the truth. (p. 341)

He suggests that narratives highlight the ways in which stories help people make sense of their lives and that the constructivist teaches clients "that narratives have a beginning (a historical context), a middle (the present situations), and an end (a hoped-for projection of ourselves into the future)" (p. 342). He suggests the use of journal narratives that are often read to the group and that reflect the developing story they write about themselves and the group as a whole. This tends to facilitate cohesion according to Brower, and helps them develop a shared narrative. He suggests role-play as another useful technique, permitting members to practice new roles. This becomes a laboratory in which members are urged to draw parallels between their feelings and actions in and out of the group.

While Brower's work is a reflection of the narrative approach, there are elements that suggest too much remains of the positivist or modernist approaches to helping. The first is the expertness of the worker, who he refers to as "leader." (It is generally better to save that term for the person in the group who is the group's leader, that is, president, chairperson, even informal leader). The leader "provides guidelines," sets the agenda, establishes the rules, and so forth. These are tasks that in social group work, the worker understands is only partially his/her responsibility and is the "work" of the group. In addition, there is a structured "phase" theory process. It is never clear in stage theory where one phase ends and another begins. This is an attempt to be scientific, but ambiguities exist, and individual differences are ignored.

Most of the work done in narrative has been in the tradition of verbal therapy, that is, the "talking cure." As the ideas of narrative have spread, attempts to use it differently have evolved. Zimmerman and Shepherd (1993) have used art therapy and letter writing in their work with groups of bulimic women. The authors note that group therapy is an effective treatment for Bulimia. At the beginning sessions of the group, members were asked to name the negative influences of Bulimia. Some of the names included "Amoeba"; "Werewolf, as if I'm changed into something horrible"; Helga, a German woman who "pushes food on me, even when I am full." They would discuss these names in the group. "Members would cry as they expressed how the bulimia affected their lives and laugh at the descriptions of the bulimia influences" (pp. 26–28).

> In addition to White's conversational technique, drawing pictures of the externalized force, a visual representation enhanced the externalization process . . . Amoeba looked like the face of a hairy monster . . . Werewolf was an abstract picture entitled, transformation. . . . Following the naming and drawing exercises, the group was given a homework assignment. Each member was asked to write a letter to the external influence. (p. 280)

The authors have found the combination of program media with conversation as a very effective method of empowering clients.

Once again we see the worker modifying narrative in a very creative way. The worker leads from his/her strengths. However, giving homework puts the power in the hands of the worker, and homework may also remind people of a class and childhood. It might have been better for the worker to ask what they might do to carry with them some of the positive experience the session had provided. Did they think anyone might like to see the pictures? Who might and who might not care to see them? Do they think their "external influence" might want to see them? Why or why not? Conversations about the exercise would also be interesting. How did they feel about the exercise? Why did they think it was done? What would they think of a homework assignment? How would homework make them feel about the worker? These are not presented as a barrage of questions, but as part of a give and take conversation.

In the following group record we observe a group of women who had been battered.

W: Isn't it interesting that your son didn't get mad and curse the police, but that he is abusive to you? Do you think he learned that somewhere?

L: Yeah, he learned it at home.

F. Definitely, they know to whom they can be abusive they get it from their fathers.

L: Oh yeah, I know my son knows when to manipulate me.

W: Is it the same way your husband did?

L: I think so.

F: Unfortunately, the children suffer the same abuse as us. Then they do it to others.

W: I wonder if this abusive behavior is something your husband/ partners learned from somebody?

L: I think so. I think they probably learned from their home. I read a funny article about the 1950s, women were told how to take care of their husbands when they come home from work. Keep the children quiet: things should be picked up. It was funny at first but then . . .

I: There were times my mom told me how to be a good wife.

W: Do you think it's something in the culture?
Some of the women laughed.

I: My husband's mother still tells me what to do.

L: You should tell her not to.

I: don't think I can, I just get angry.

Y: What are you afraid of?

I: I don't know, she's an old lady, 78 years old.

L: You should tell her.

W: What keeps you from saying something?

I: I am afraid to.

W. What do the rest of you think?

Y: Mothers-in-laws can scare you, I know.

L: I always said what I wanted to say, that's why I have trouble with my husband. When I don't let him abuse me he gets into a temper tantrum.

W: I, does fear keep you from confronting your husband too?

I: It used to, but he has gotten calmer, particularly since he knows I come here. He still gets angry, The other day he didn't like what I said, and he broke the cell phone, but he didn't hit me

W: So you overcame your fear, and stood up for yourself?
I: Yes.
L: That's great
W: Did you feel good?
I: Yes, but his anger still scares me.

The meeting continued, and the women spoke more about the group
and how helpful it had been to them, and how they felt liberated. We will
look at just one more section:

F: I got tired of being afraid and living the way I lived.
W: How do you feel now?
F: I feel great. I feel liberated, free.

An example of a group (author unknown) of sexually victimized children illustrates how a group member can help with the deconstruction
process. The discussion is with a mother whose boyfriend had abused the
children. The older daughter has started to hit her younger sisters. The
mother has just called her a tyrant:

Worker: Does she remind you of anyone?
Angela: No. I was never like that. She's way too bossy for her age.
Sharon: Maybe she learned from your first husband . . . I mean your
         husband.
Angela: She started it after we left. She hasn't seen him for a long
         time. Could she have?
Worker: It's possible, especially if she's trying to be the daddy. What
         goes through your mind when you're mad at her? What
         words?
Angela: You can't tell me what to do! You can't talk like that!
Worker: Have you ever wanted to say that to anyone else?
Angela: Her . . . and my father. I would have said that to him if I
         could. He did some really mean things. Cruel. She's cruel,
         too, like him. (looks sad, defeated)
Worker: Do you have the same feelings for each of them?
Angela: I think so . . . Mad . . . and hopeless. She makes me feel that
         way again.
Worker: So when you try to be a parent and tell her what to do, you
         feel all your old kid feelings?
Angela: Yes. When it's a fight, I feel hopeless with her.

In this brief episode we see the worker and another group member work at constructing a new narrative by searching out some of the blanks in Angela's story. There is also an effort at what can be seen as externalizing the problem of hopelessness, or "old kid feelings." Questions could follow to search out the unique experience, when in spite of feeling hopeless her efforts at being a parent were successful. One of the worker's questions caused Angela to look back and see when the hitting began. There can be some follow-up on this. Did she as a child take over some of her mother's role? What are her feelings about the separation and her letting the daughter take over?

Other group members might be involved in discussing how they parent, what works, and so on. We don't know from this record whether or not the daughter is being served in any way, but we would want to find out and see what help she might be willing to accept. If this were a family group, then it would be possible to use a circular question approach where each of the family members would be asked for their view of the situation.

The matter of empowerment has become an important issue in the profession. Most models of helping are currently focused on strength perspectives rather than deficits. This is a particularly important matter when working with minority and other oppressed groups in our society. Rasheed and Rasheed (1999) point out some of the need and the difficulties in group work with African-American men. One of the approaches they suggest is the provision of an Afrocentric base in the practice. More specifically, one suggestion is based on Dr. Maulana Karenga's principles of NguZo Saba. Dr. Karenga was the originator and force behind the evolution of the African-American celebration called Kwanzaa (Karenga, 1998). The celebration of this holiday has gained international observance and increased self pride.

RE-MEMBERING: THE HEALING STORIES OF THE PAST

White, in some of his training sessions, has discussed the work of Barbara Myerhoff (1982) who worked with the frail elderly in Venice, California. The group with whom she met was made up primarily of Jewish holocaust survivors. This was a cohort group that shared some important similarities. Meyerhoff points out that,

Sometimes conditions conspire to make a generational cohort acutely self-conscious and then they become active participants in their own history

and provide their own sharp, instant definitions of themselves and explanations for their destiny, past and future. They are then knowing actors in
a historical drama they script, rather than subjects in someone else's study.
They "make" themselves, sometimes even "make themselves up," an activity which is not only inevitable or automatic but reserved for special people and special circumstances. It is an artificial and exhilarating undertaking, this self-construction. (Meyerhoff, 1982, p. 104)

She discusses the importance of their telling the memories of their
childhoods. The memories served to be collected as moral documents
which preserved their past. At special occasions, some of their re-membered
stories were presented in front of their families.

> A story told aloud to progeny or peers is, of course more than a text. It is an
> event. When it is presented presentationally, its effect on the listener is
> profound, and the latter, if more than a mere passive receiver or validator.
> The listener is changed.
>
> When the sessions were at their best, the old people were conscious of
> the importance of their integration work, not only for themselves but for
> posterity, however modestly represented. Then they felt the high satisfac-
> tion of being able to fulfill themselves as individuals as Exemplars of a tra-
> dition at once. (Myerhoff, p. 111)

It is easy to see why White sees the work of Myerhoff as closely related
to what he is trying to do in Narrative Therapy. There is not only a clear
picture of the importance of stories in the lives of persons, but also the
construction of stories that have preferred meaning. In addition, there is
the presentation of the new life story to an audience and its importance
as self-sustaining. She sees narratives as ". . . strategies that provide opportunities for being seen on one's own terms, garnering witnesses to one's
worth, vitality and being" (Myerhoff, 1982, p. 263). Myerhoff's works
deal with the importance of meaning in the person's life, particularly relevant in working with the elderly, and is well worth becoming familiar
with. It demonstrates the importance of group interactions and their relationships with others and themselves.

In their book on narrative therapy, Freedman and Combs (1996) note
just two examples of narrative with groups. Putting aside whether the
family is considered a group or not, clearly at the early stages of its use it
was seen as part of Family Therapy. They suggest that the group offers
people an opportunity to become the audience to each other (p. 255).
This seems to be a major function of the group in their view. They quote
the work of Adams-Westcott and Isenbart (1995).

We invite group members to develop connections and create a community that supports each participant's personal journey of change. This "community" provides an audience to: (1) develop their own self-knowledge; (2) practice more validating stories about self; and (3) incorporate preferred narratives into their lived experience. (p. 335)

They also cite the work of Laube and Trefz (1994),

The group participants are the initial audience for the telling of stories in a safe setting where there is validation, commonality, affirmation about how depression has been a dominant influence. The members help each other transfer their tales by being an audience for discovering exceptions and noticing differences. (p. 33)

An interesting use of narrative with a couples group, in which one partner has a history of child sexual abuse, was reported by Adams-Westcott and Isenbart (1995). It was not clear whether the participants were currently involved in an abusive relationship. The authors experimented with a variety of formats: 12 week, 90-minute groups, and a 6-session, 2½-hour structured workshop. When possible, they used female and male therapists working together to facilitate the sessions. Couples were invited to introduce themselves and share the stories about how they became partners. "The therapists arrived at the first meeting with a list of candidate goals, and asked the participants for their ideas about how the group could be useful to them." (p. 17)

This helped create the agenda, and they were then given a series of exercises. It is interesting to note how much direction came from the workers, starting with deciding in advance the number of sessions, the structure of each meeting, and the exercises to be used. Attempts were made to modify exercises and the process of the meetings in keeping with the wishes of the group, but clearly there was a great deal that was pre-set. Although the language used seemed to infer choices on the part of the participants, one might wonder what Foucault might think of this statement, "At the beginning of each session participants were *invited* to evaluate the ideas discussed the previous week. This brief *ritual* served several purposes" (p. 24, italics added). The use of the term invited might suggest a choice, but is it? The term "ritual" reveals a structured approach to the meetings, which set the direction, at least for a large part of the session. While rituals are important and recognized as so by the narrativists (Epston and White), ritualization, which suggests a rigid format, can close out room for participatory decisions. Change of content might be very difficult, particularly in the 6-session group, where challenging the leadership might be seen as threatening the life of the group by some members. One might ask how this fits with the idea that the worker is not the expert, and the narrative philosophy that there should be a minimal amount of worker authority and use of power. The answer seems to lie in their modification of the narrative approach in their workshops. In discussing one of the major exercises that they used, they note that the conceptual model of some questions was influenced by the solution-focused approach. We are reminded of Michael White's caution that narrative cannot be tacked on to other approaches—it is not a series of techniques, but a philosophy of helping.

Couples who participated reported positive change, as did the referring professionals. They reported that the 12-week format would have permitted them to feel more comfortable and share more of their lives. The authors also note that previous participants were willing to attend meetings and serve as consultants to members of future groups. They felt that the most notable changes were in their sense of mastery. This included advocacy for themselves and others to challenge the conditions that contribute to victimization.

Miska Lysak (1995) discusses the use of narrative with incarcerated teenagers. "Consultation groups (involving teenagers and parents who are in or have completed therapy) are also used to advise the therapist on the effects of the therapy and to suggest ways of enhancing the process" (p. 3).

GROUPS AND COMMUNITY ACTION

At a meeting in Los Angeles in the late 1990s, Michael White spoke briefly about a group called Power to Our Journeys, with which he had been working in Australia. He then proceeded to help raise money for the group by selling shirts, which he had brought with him. While his work with the group was innovative and exciting, his commitment to the welfare of the group was inspiring. Here was a person that not only talked the talk, but also walked the walk.

An account of the group's experiences written by the members notes that, "The Power of Our Journeys meetings provide a forum for us to talk about many of the experiences of life" (Bridgitte, 1996). It goes on to point out how the many therapists they have seen over the years and who have generally given them a diagnosis of schizophrenia, have refused to acknowledge their experiences with voices and visions. "Needless to say, this silencing has profoundly negative consequences on all our lives. All of us have felt abandoned because of this. It has been important for us to experience our work, to reclaim our lives from the troublesome voices and visions as a struggle against injustice." The article details some of the work that the group had to do to arrive at the point where they were able to change their lives significantly and noted particularly the work of White. The group also speaks of their logo, which depicts Mount Kilimanjaro. One of the members who had climbed that mountain remarked that getting her life back from the hostile voices was a journey that was not dissimilar to the climb to the top of Mount Kilimanjaro. "It is hard work," she said, "but with the right preparations and provisions, a good map of the terrain, access to forecasts that make it possible to predict the weather ahead, and the appropriate support systems, it can be done" (pp. 12–13).

This group, which met at the Dulwich Center in Adelaide, Australia, has become an advocate for others like themselves, and has tried to develop alternative materials that could be sent to various libraries in psychiatric hospitals. These could serve as examples along with standard texts. Here is a good example of how a program that starts out with clinical implications starts to evolve a story that includes impacting the social forces of which it is a part, and which to a degree subjugated it.

The worker in community organization is often seen by the group as the "leader." This evolves from the process which often begins with the worker recruiting and organizing persons in the community on behalf of some activity. As the group evolves its own structure and leadership, the worker starts to act more as a consultant. This, however, is not always a simple shift in role.

At a meeting with a landlord who has been negligent in keeping the apartment in decent shape the worker confronted the landlord and took the leadership for most of the meeting. The tenants, all women, when asked by the landlord to say what they were upset with him about, were unable to respond. The landlord agreed to some changes but only after the worker made strong demands on him. Following the meeting, the worker and the tenants gathered to discuss the next step. The worker discussed the meeting and said that from now on the group would have to start taking on more responsibility. One of the members said, "But Joe, you are our leader, we are nothings without you." Some of the other members shouted their agreement.

This is not unusual. In a sense, the members become dependent on the worker and it is difficult for the group to develop its own leadership, particularly when the worker is effective and/or well liked. It is important for the worker not to be the one who speaks for the group, but that the group members become empowering and their own agents.

One example of the misuse of power of the worker with a group is illustrated by the following statement by a worker who is developing a therapy group from clients she has seen previously on an individual basis. "Since each of the women had been seeing me in individual or family therapy for various presenting problems previous to the group work, all reported 'trusting' me in knowing what 'would work' therapeutically for each of them" (Gagerman, 1997). Can one really understand others, can one understand oneself sufficiently to know what other people need?

One of the ways in which the expertise and power of the worker can be used most constructively without hindering the group's growth is for the worker to take on the role of "Instructed Advocate" (Abels, 1971). An instructed advocate is a social worker whose advocacy is defined and limited by the group with which he/she works, and whose major task is to work with the community in its efforts to bring about environmental change. It is the story of a community wanting to re-author the situation in which they find themselves. In this case, the common re-authoring project was to change the living conditions for the tenants in a particular housing unit. The agreements that get worked out between the members and the worker reflect just when the worker will be the advocate, under what conditions, and when the group members will be their own advocates, and that the worker will not speak "for" the group without mutual agreements as to the context and the content. An important part of the agreements deal with the development of the group's own leadership.

White has started to make some use of narrative practice in the community organization arena. Stephen Madigan (1996), from the Yaletown Family Therapy, has noticed that many of the discourses his clients share have been individualized and that there is a need for more community discourse. He hopes for an externalization of internalized community discourse. He calls for the therapists to take a more active position politically—it is a call to radicalize the profession (Madigan, 1996). If therapists were to heed that call, we might soon see more efforts to work with groups and organize communities. This can be done within the narrative framework without the worker taking over the direction of the group. The work of the "Power to Our Journeys" group attests to that possibility. Below are some comments about how they see themselves.

> How did we get together? It was our experiences of narrative therapy that provided the basis for our connection with each other. . . . We get together

once a month, and invite Michael White to join us to keep a special record of our conversation and to ask questions that assist us to express our thoughts on various issues. After each of these meetings, Michael puts together our ideas in a document which serves as a record of our evolving knowledges and of the development in our skills of living. . . . This group has played a very significant part in rekindling our love for life, and in assisting us to achieve a quality of life that we could never have predicted . . .

Michael has proposed that the libraries of psychiatric hospitals be obliged to include the sort of alternative texts that might be created by collections of the sort of therapeutic documents that we provide examples of here . . . these alternative texts just might be more helpful to people who are struggling with troublesome voices and visions than the standard texts. (Brigitte, Sue, Mem, and Veronika, pp. 11–16)

Here we see how a group which began as a therapeutic group re-authored themselves, not only individually, but also as a group. They change the story from a group seeking help from others, to a group offering help to others, doing social action and attempting to influence their environment and serve as a mutual-aid resource.

VIRTUAL GROUPS AND AUDIENCES

While most of White and Epston's (1990) work focuses on individuals and families, their efforts to incorporate others into the situation are an important element of their work. This includes the creation of virtual groups by bringing them into the consciousness of the client and is a particularly cogent and significant part of their practice approach.

The endurance of new stories, as well as their elaboration, is enhanced if there is an audience to their performance. There is a dual aspect to this. First, in the act of witnessing such performances, the audience contributes to the writing of new meanings, and this has real effects on the audience's interactions with the story's subjects. Second, when the subjects of the story read the audience's experience of the new performance, either through speculation about these experiences or by more direct identification, they engage in revisions and extensions of the new stories. (p. 114)

These are dealt with through conversations and or letters that help participants reflect on how others might see their newly evolved stories, and the changes that they have made. In essence they create an audience in the mind of the client. These may be considered virtual groups and can serve as reference points for decision making. Their use of certificates and diplomas serves a similar purpose. The person creates a virtual organization in their mind that is giving them these awards.

CONCLUSION

While there is a great deal of theory in narrative related to the importance of groups, it has not yet been reflected by much actual application in the field. Many of the authors have used the group as an audience, or as a support group for the person who was being helped. None of the authors reflect on the fact that the family is a group, and therefore very little attention is paid to group dynamics and the impact on the participants of the interactions among members.

Another important item that needs to be considered in working with groups is where the worker positions him/herself. If the worker becomes the central figure, then the group will continually look to him or her. The group's own leadership and creative ideas will become subservient to those of the worker who will soon be seen as the expert or the person with all the answers. We are not suggesting that it is necessary to develop a contract, but that the worker's actions must convey the idea that the members must use each other and help each other as much as possible. In a sense, the worker demands that the rewriting of the narrative is the work of the participants. There may be a little editing and plot thickening that the worker does, but it is the members' story, albeit that the worker may be a character in the plot. Dean suggests that the traditional hierarchical relationship between the worker and the group be avoided and a more collaborative relationship developed, with the worker more like a participant observer. The worker takes a learner's stance and influence moves in both directions between client and worker. She notes, however, that the

> group leader is also responsible for managing the conversation. 'Managing' means seeing that all members are engaged and it means creating openings in which their stories can be told. The group leader may ask questions that expand stories, call on members to respond to one another's stories, clarify the different possible meaning of stories and intervene in ways that help people change their stories. (Dean, 1998, p. 35)

Dean's comments on the role of the worker reflect a major difficulty in working with groups, the matter of worker control. Although she attempts to narrow down the amount of direction that should come from the worker, she is stuck with the word manager and attempts to limit its interpretation. She has the managing, however, coming from the worker and not from the group. A major effort of the worker is for the group to assume most of the role she is assigning to the worker, who by the way she refers to as the "leader." This, of course, is common usage, but in itself places the direction in the hands of the worker. The "leader" is the person(s) in the group who is given or takes leadership. It may be an elected officer, the person the group talks to or, the person who talks the most. In fact, in different group situations different members might take over the leadership of the group. If the worker is also the leader, then often the group's leadership has been stifled or the group is not developing in a way that allows it to do its own re-authoring and is dependent on the worker as "editor."

A major use of the group as a helping tool has been in the use of the reflective team. Due to the efforts of White and others, the function of the reflecting team and the nature of their feedback has changed in ways that have made the reflecting team more helpful to the clients, rather than as advice to the helper as to how to proceed, or illustrating where they went wrong. It has turned more into a support group and a reflective opportunity for the client than a critique.

As a final illustration, we will look at how the group helps both its members and the worker to do a better job. The example is of a boys group, 10–11 year olds, formed by a school to discuss the problems they are having at school. The group has been meeting for a few months and one of the children, Pete in particular, is having a difficult time. He has been a problem in the group and at times they have wanted him out, but they have come to accept his wild behavior over time. At this meeting Pete has admitted he can't read well, and if he could, maybe he would do better at school. They are talking about a reading/ learning class that might be helpful to him, and the other boys tell him that he should take it.

Pete: "OK how can I get in?" The group offered suggestions, and the worker said "Would you like me to find out the information?" He said yes, but the worker notes that he seemed hesitant. "You're really not sure, Pete?" The others heard this and asked why, Pete responded, "the school will put me in 101." "The group told me that this was the dumbest class." The boys agreed that they might. I asked Pete if he was afraid to be in that class, and that he might be called dumb? He said, "Yeah." The others said, "You've got to be afraid of that." I asked, "You all afraid of that?" They said they were. A few said they didn't think they would put him back: "Not if you're just asking for help." The others said I should find out first, without mentioning his name. (the author of this record unknown)

The group not only supports Pete and suggests ways he might get help, as does the worker, but it has information she doesn't have about "that" reading class, and even suggests how she might go about getting information for Pete without putting him in jeopardy.

It is important to use the group to help. Each of the members is expected to use themselves, not only for their own well-being, but as helpers as well. The ability to give to others is extremely important, particularly for those who have seen themselves as always needing help from others and not giving back in return. The power of being helpful increases the person's sense of him/herself as an agent of change, but also the feeling of their own self-worth.

8

Supportive Approaches and Mutual Aid

> Americans of all ages, all conditions, and all dispositions constantly form associations. . . . The Americans make associations to give entertainment, to found seminaries, to build inns, to construct churches, to diffuse books. . . . Wherever at the end of some new undertaking you see the government in France, or a man of rank in England, in the United States, you are sure to find an association.
>
> Alexis de Tocqueville

A major purpose of the social work profession is to help people make connections with each other and with their social institutions. It is the variety and complexity of role relationships that enrich people's lives. A major means by which these aims are accomplished is by the enhancement of mutual aid and social support. This might take place on a small group scale or community wide (Caplan, 1974; Katz, 1993; Whittaker & Garbarino, 1983).

The history of mutual aid associations predates any formal welfare system in the United States. They included burial societies, insurance organizations, and health support groups, all aimed at giving some type of benefit to their members. Over a hundred years before there was social security, there were mutual benefit associations. These groups existed among most ethnic and religious groups. They often served as sources of survival during times of extreme need. Their development and their demise are ably discussed in David T. Beito's book, *From Mutual Aid to the Welfare State* (Beito, 2000).

While many of the original functions of those mutual aid organizations, particularly those aspects requiring large amount of funds, ended with the coming of social security, the spirit of mutual aid survives. There is a growing recognition of the importance of support groups as an adjunct and at times as a major force for individual and social change. Regardless of the situation that persons find themselves in, including mental illness, divorce, loss of a family member, unemployment, widowhood, alcoholism, child abuse, obesity, depression, or chronic illness; whether they are nine or ninety; whether it is the stress of neighborhood change; the stress of the holocaust, from individual concern to national catastrophe; there is a growing understanding that social support is a buffer against the stresses of those situations and countless others.

By social support we mean the human, emotional, informational, and/or the material supports provided by kin, friends, peers, neighbors, service providers, and others with whom one has an ongoing relationship and to whom one can turn in times of need.

Self-help is the voluntary joining of persons with similar life-stress concerns into small groups (at times a section of a national group) whose purpose is mutual aid and/or the accomplishment of social change related to that concern, such as Mothers Against Drunk Driving (MADD). Katz defines self-help more formally as:

Voluntary small group structures for mutual aid of a special purpose. They are usually formed by the peers who have come together for mutual assistance in satisfying a common need, overcoming a common handicap or life disrupting problem, and bringing about desired social and/or personal change. The initiators and members of such groups perceive that their needs are not or can not be met by and through existing social institutions. (Katz, 1970)

One of the important tasks for the worker in the narrative approach is to help the client make use of whatever community support is available. While this may mean creating support groups, it also means helping the person become involved in the community. Narrative therapists make use of celebrations, certificates, and all types of ceremonies to bring the person into the changing landscape. Many of the ideas related to the ceremonies and rites of passage, which White discusses, have come from Epston's background in Anthropology. Part of the letter writing ideas are also ethnographic types of recording. This, combined with the Anthropologist's training and beliefs about maintaining the integrity of the studied group's culture, is reflected in the "know-nothing" philosophy and anti-expert philosophy of narrative practice.

During crisis situations, such as hurricanes, earthquakes, and floods, there is an expectation that community members will rally to help each other, often at great risk to their own lives. When the most dramatic, dangerous aspect of the hurricane is over they will share their shelter, offer comfort, and support to their neighbors. At times, as in the recent earthquake in Turkey where forty thousand people died, nations come to help and offer support. This is even true in cases where the countries are hostile to each other like Turkey and Cyprus, or like the United States and North Korea were, where food is given when a famine occurs. No one makes these people do what they are doing, yet there seems to be a universal convention that everyone will help. It is at these times that we see the idea of mutual aid at its finest.

The idea is a simple one; people help each other overcome the difficulties of life that they are often not able to handle on their own, or can handle better if there are others who can aid in the helping. There is no expectation of external rewards other than the expectation that this natural helping process will be returned if necessary.

Once we get past the crisis, however, there is growing evidence that the culture in our country during the past decade has increasingly turned from concern for others to self-indulgence. The bottom line has become a major element in the thinking of the younger generation. And a number of authors have discussed the loss of meaning that young people are feeling. Some have seen this as a root cause of alienation and disrespect for others, leading at times to serious incidents in which young people seek attention by heinous deeds.

Reports following the Littleton, Colorado school killings by two teenage boys suggest that it might have been related in part to this sense of meaninglessness and isolation that some of the young people felt. They were seen as odd, discounted by their peers, and those adults who were in a position to be helpful to them, including teachers, and counselors who did not seem to notice their isolation and their need to make connections. The connections that they did make were with others who were isolated too and felt a lack of meaning in their lives. For many, high school is but a stepping stone to a career, to college, or to wealth. This has become a general requirement to be accepted as a total person. Not making a fortune by forty means you are a failure. The values of our society have been shifting, and while our practice has been shifting with it, it has not shifted in a direction that would counter some of the shortcomings of an alienated people, but rather is subject to the same desire to be a success, which in our culture now means wealthy, which in helping means therapy, and particularly private practice.

Our multitudinous and evolving approaches to helping have not recognized that this cultural shift requires a practice shift that helps people move less to a "me" centered life, but to a shared existence based on positive and equal connections with others. Historically, that has been one of the major strengths of social group work, the value of the group, the community, and the benefits of mutual aid.

In the field of social work, the contributions of William Schwartz stand out, particularly his contributions to the development of the interactive or mediating model in social group work. His belief that the worker was the mediator between the needs of society and the needs of the client was an important step in furthering the understanding of the importance of social forces in providing a context for change (Schwartz, 1961). His work developed the ideas first proposed by Bertha Reynolds (1965) in her work, particularly in her book *Between Community and the Client*. One of the ideas, which Schwartz expanded on, was the role of mutual aid as a factor in social group work. It recognized that the worker need not be an expert, and that there was power in the group to help itself. Schwartz might very well be seen as the first postmodernist in social work. He actively worked at deconstructing the social work myths of his day, and was concerned about the focus on individualism as well as the foibles of the profession, and was certainly in the forefront in seeing the value of self-help and mutual aid groups.

Schwartz (1961) reviewed the history of the idea of people aiding each other, noting the work of Kropotkin who traced the biological roots of mutual aid in animals and human beings for the benefit of their societies and mutual aid from insect and animal behavior to the building of community. Schwartz noted:

> The group is an enterprise in mutual aid, an alliance of individuals who need each other in varying degrees to work on certain common problems. The important fact is a helping system in which the clients need each other as well as the worker. This need to use each other, to create not one but many helping relationships, is a vital part of the group process and constitutes a common need over and above the specific task for which the group was formed. (1961, p. 19)

In keeping with these ideas, White has always noted that the client is the worker's best consultant. He does not have any problem suggesting that the client bring others to the session, either as support or as a person who might be helpful in the process, for example, to translate language or cultural beliefs to the worker.

Schulman points out how this advances the help given to the client:

> This conceptualization of the group as a mutual aid system had profound implications for the role of the worker leading the group. Rather than seeing one's role as providing help within a group context, the worker would concentrate on the tasks involved in strengthening the members' ability to help each other. The worker in this view, is but one source of help to clients. (Schulman, 1984, p. 52)

This fits in nicely with the narrative perspective of minimizing the control of the worker and he/she being seen as an expert. There are many workers in the mutual aid group. In fact, part of the role of the worker is to help all the members contribute. It also enhances the sense of power that the members have.

The following is an excerpt from a self-help group for arthritis patients. They are confronting a doctor about what they have gotten from the group.

> "No doctor, that's not it at all. It's just that seeing her courage gives me courage." This was a lady who would not have dreamed of contradicting her doctor before. The group really let him know he was way off the mark. And he took it very well.
>
> The worker notes, "Before the group, I don't think anyone of them would have dared disagree. They would have just sat there and listened and discounted their own experience if it was in conflict with his. But now they stand up for what they know. It's been quite impressive to see how the power of the group has grown. So has the way they insist on doing things for each other." (Riesman, pp. 79–80)

Recent studies have found that mutual aid may reflect some of the Darwinian ideas related to evolution. It was in those societies in which members aided each other that survival of the group was enhanced. The numbers of people in the clans were small, and groups needed each member, in order to maintain the crucial minimum to maintain themselves. This idea of mutual aid runs contrary to the belief that each person was in competition with the other for the scarce resources and that the weak were left on their own.

In social group work, the theme was that members of a group could help each other, and helping was related to the contributions of each member that added to the power of the group as a helping tool. It was the group process that was a unique contribution to the helping arena, and the major practice approach which distinguishes it from other work which involves groups in some way. It was in the last fifty or so years that those therapeutic groups have gained wide acceptance. The more traditional helping models such as psychoanalytic therapists were reluctant and often clearly hostile to the turning from the one-to-one models to the use of the group. While there were some valiant therapists who saw the value in working with groups, such as Slavson and Ackerman, few Freudian analysts ventured into the group work arena, and even among them it was more of an individual treatment model in front of the group. The understanding and use of the group process to help was not clearly understood or utilized.

Mutual aid is a process in which persons help each other to achieve mutually acceptable goals. While it is often used within the group, the growth of support groups has shown that the idea of mutual aid can often incorporate strangers who are willing to share in the helping process. Part of the expansion of the in-group mutual aid ideas to broader support groups came from the work of people with special problems, often organized by relatives of a person who needed aid, such as children with disabilities. Currently the major support/mutual aid group is Alcoholics Anonymous (AA). The recognition of the importance of the group for change and the need for a person to make connections with it at a time of need is most clearly understood by observing AA's popularity and its international recognition. It has served as a model for other problems in addition to alcohol, such as drugs and gambling. A great deal has been written about these efforts and there is no need to examine how they operate at this point, other than to note that most often they are not led by professionals in the helping field, and are often led by persons who are recovering from the concern that the group is dealing with.

Narrative practice is an approach to mutual aid that is a little different. One of the uses is the reflective team that we will take up at another chapter in the text. The second is the use of the "virtual group."

Imagine what you might be called on to do if you were working with a client who had a unique illness that he/she was recovering from and that no one else in the area suffered from similarly. You are aware of people in other cities, states, or even countries that have had a similar problem and are recovered or recovering. You might create a "fan club" and ask some of those people to write or call occasionally; or if you had clients of your own who had similar problems they might call or write telling of how they overcame such problems, or to watch out for the tricks that "sneaky poo" might try, that he is a very sly character.

What if there were no clients or others around that might be useful as a support network? Would it be in the best interest of the client to make

up a support group? For example, Epston and White (1990) have offered
certificates or degrees from artificial Universities that they create. In
order to graduate, the person must pass certain requirements such as two
or three letters from members of the family that they have indeed accomplished certain steps in the process of healing, whether by obtaining
references of change or by accomplishing some tasks. While there is definitely an element of expert direction in these kinds of "set ups," the purpose is to be helpful to the client. Clearly, a postmodern view would
attest that no model is ideal or perfect.

I am reminded of the groups built around homebound children so
that they would have an opportunity to be involved with other children.
One of the first and most creative of these programs was developed by
Ralph Kolodny in Boston about fifty years ago. Clearly, these were not
natural groups in that they were not friends, neighbors, or knew the child,
but their importance lay in the need of contact with others for the development of the child. It led to an unusual type of "friendship" group.

Epston and White (1990) have used such approaches of connecting individual clients with their families and with others, by using former clients,
current clients, members of the community and organizations, sometimes
fictitious, designed to lend support and the power of mutual aid. They constantly try to make connections with others who might have positive views of
the clients, past or present. At times, ideas of people no longer alive, but
important to the client's story, are brought into the helping conversation.

In one exciting program, White (1995a) makes use of the experiences
of women who have left their husbands, to research the stages that take
place as they go through the process. He suggests that crossing borders is
an appropriate metaphor, which makes the difficulties vivid. The person
crossing to a new land has initial fears as the decision is being made with
hopes of the new land, realities of being an immigrant and a stranger and
sometimes returning to the "old country" but sometimes settling in.
White uses the common experiences of the women, with their permission, to plot their experiences on a graph. He has plotted points on the trip
in which there are both highs and lows. These are discussed with the new
client who may be about to embark on that journey, see where they are,
and view the total possible landscape. The importance of these connections with others is that they act as a strong element of support.

He says,

> I regularly encourage the women who are consulting me to mark where
> they think they are on the journey. Their mark helps them see the trajectory

called a "Migration of Identity." The very act of doing so brings about a dramatic change in their attitude towards what they are going through . . . (1995, p. 102)

He might say, "This is where Jane was at the three-way mark, you are three weeks into this, where are you?" They might say they are feeling better or worse off than Jane. Sometimes women who have made the trip are called in to talk to the new voyager. This permits them to anticipate some of the bumpy roads, and helps them feel that many others are in the same boat. He notes that planning a celebration at the journey's end can also assist in reestablishing connections with others. It is also a process of involvement; the client does the planning, sends out invitations, and so forth.

Every effort is made to develop a support group when it seems important to do so. White believes it is important to combat any *abuse* teams that the client might have with a *nurturing* team. He often lists himself as the first member of the club.

THE IMPORTANCE OF CONNECTIONS

The understanding that in the natural course of growing up children need to make connections with others, usually peers of the same age, was an important factor in the creation of the groups for the homebound as well as the "virtual groups" that White and Epston make use of. While it might be better to have real live peers for the person who is being helped, this is not always possible. With adults, some of the 12-Step programs do provide the contacts if people wish to use them, and usually with people who have been in the same boat.

One of the important problems that workers have to deal with adults is the feeling of loneliness that many of them have. This is true for older people who are alone because of the death of a spouse or partner or because their children have all left home. The job of the worker with these adults calls for helping them make connections with other people, and the use of community resources is of importance in this area (Abels & Abels, 1980). No artificial group would make sense. The use of the chat rooms on the computer and the computer itself offers one way for the person to connect with others. The use of the computer and the Internet can be helpful, but needs further exploration. Some authors have dealt with this area and have reported success. Whether or not loneliness can be overcome satisfactorily is still an issue under consideration. But for a number of people it may be one of the only ways that they can maintain connections with the reality of other people, their views and their interest in them, even though it may be a person whom they never meet. For a number of years it was very clear that some of the radio talk shows served that purpose for people who had no one to talk to. They became regulars on some of the programs, calling nightly, to the extent that the disk jockey became familiar with them and would expect a call, and they could relate to him/her on a first name basis. Television has not provided similar opportunities, but the Internet has.

In the group situation, narrative provides additional opportunities for connections to be made. If the story that the group re-authors for itself includes being helpful as a group to the members, then they may provide connections outside of the group situation, as well, which helps in the mutual aid process (Adams-Wescott & Denbart, 1995). Frequently the worker has seen the group as a tool only when it meets.

One of the most interesting and inspiring efforts of mutual aid is reflected in the mobilization by the gay community to organize on their own behalf around the AIDS epidemic. At first, the reaction of the general community to the plight of HIV victims was to ignore it, belittle it, and attack it as a gay disease. Very little was being done by the general community to develop services or to organize national efforts to deal with the problem. While many populations suffered from AIDS, it was the mobilization by gays that started to make the general community notice what was going on and to lend its support, influence the politicians, and combat the forces that felt AIDS was an appropriate punishment for "deviant" sexual activity.

Were it not for the ability and motivation of the gay community, the cures that are now on the market would have been delayed even further than they have been. This lack of concern by the community was another example of Foucault's and narrative's theoretical position, that certain groups are seen as more worthy than others and those in power will control how those groups are treated. It was only through a counteruse of power, both economic and moral, that the gay community was able to demand a more enlightened and forward looking policy related to AIDS. It reflected some of Moreno's thinking in his book, *Who Shall Survive*, that those who could count on strong networks were more likely to survive (Moreno, 1934).

The work of Rhodes and Brown (1991) on resilience offers some evidence that connection plays an important role in children's ability to survive. Garbarino's work (Garbarino, Kosteiny, & Dubroy, 1991) supports a similar view.

CONCLUSION

In a paper presented in 1980, the authors, reflecting on the works of Jennings and Moreno, wrote that they believed, "A major focus of social group work ought to be the strengthening and development of social networks. This is a relevant assignment for group work because of the extent of social discontinuity and group work's historical participatory orientation" (Abels & Abels, 1980). This was before AIDS, before the Gay and Lesbian equality movements, before HMOs, and before the Internet. We see no reason to believe that the focus should change. In fact, enabling such networks might be considered a major purpose of the profession.

The support network has become a universally recognized way of dealing with some of the stressors that impact the clients we work with. While this support network is often made up of family members, chronic long-term illness often places extreme stress on the caretakers, who can lose control of their own lives. They too need some relief from their responsibilities. There are a growing number of services that give respite time to the caretakers. This is another area in which the helper has a part to play. There is a growing breakdown in family life and in neighborhoods as well as in the informal social ties (note the vanishing bank teller and computerized voices on telephones) and a growing dependency on central authorities for coordination and decision making around services. Counting on the professional for all direction, because of a lack of a network or a thin network, only increases the sense of isolation. The importance of continuity in relationships is exemplified by the fact that almost two-thirds of Holmes and Rahe's (1967) stress-causing factors are related to breaks in social continuity.

Gerald Caplan, back in 1974, noted that the individual's support system was a shield protecting him or her from dreaded psychic exposure to the complexity and disorder of modern life. The complexity has increased, and there is strong evidence that social connections have not kept pace (Putnam, 2000). The lack of connections has important ramifications for health and life expectancy.

Assuming our analysis of the current social context is fairly accurate, our professional responsibility ought to be directed toward strengthening mutual and reciprocal relationships, particularly social networks on behalf of our clients. Addressing this task contributes to the improvement of their well-being, their social arrangements, and attends to social work's historical participatory commitment, by aiding in the development of a sense of community, with others in similar situations, and with us as part of their community.

In narrative practice, mutual aid serves not only as a support to a client or group, but as a way of their developing the type of power needed to counter oppressive forces and provide some sense of camaraderie and safety as they undertake re-authoring their lives. Self-help and support groups are strong alternatives to individualist trends in society. The chat rooms on the web sites indicate how starved people are to have contact with others. We need to consider whether distance interaction is a viable alternative in the long run to helping people make contact with each other and have face-to-face support groups. It would be important to examine the effectiveness of such groups compared to the real groups with a worker present.

We close this section with a brief word on the use of the Internet and computers in general for mental health purposes. There have been studies for the past thirty years on the use of computers to do therapy (Abels, 1977b). The web sites are currently flooded with individuals and organizations offering counseling over the "net." This is a growing trend and seems to be filling an important niche. It may be that there are some persons who are more able to use help in a less face-to-face way, over the computer. It will be interesting to visualize how narrative practice would make use of the web, or if it would at all. Certainly, letters to clients could be sent by e-mail, rather than by post. This might work better for clients because of the interactive speed of e-mail.

Galinsky and Schopler (1995) have included a number of articles dealing with innovative ways to develop and use support groups. A number of articles dealing with support as well as mutual aid can also be found, with good case material in Gitterman and Shulman (1994). In a paper presented in Toronto, the authors (Abels & Abels, 2000) suggest that the development of connectedness and social connections needs to be given centrality in work with clients. Universally, research with varied populations indicates the importance of thick rather than thin connections in enhancing both mental and physical well-being.

Our final comment relates to the universal use and value of self-help, and is highlighted by a *New York Times* article illustrating its use by an entire city in Russia (Wines, 2000). By combining its forces in a self-help effort, Dubna, Russia was able to reduce its health problems and its death rates to 20% below national norms. One of the people involved in this collaborative self-help effort notes, "change is not begun without an environment that permits change" (p. 10).

9

Narrative Administration

We must go very carefully at first. The great serpent to destroy is the will to power; the desire for one man to have domain over his fellow man. Let us have no personal influence, if possible—no personal magnetism, as they used to call it, nor persuasion—no "Follow me"—but only "behold:"
(D. H. Lawrence)

The writings on narrative practice present scarce references to the pivotal role of the agency other than to refer to it as a sponsor, or the setting in which the practice is carried out. This is an odd omission for a theory which emphasizes the nature of the social context in formulating the problems that bring people for help. We also know that most of social work practice takes place within the purview of an agency. And we know as well that every program initiated has a story connected to it, which makes up a subplot in the overall agency narrative (Albert, 1987; Barry, 1997; Buss, 1989).

If we were to deconstruct these agency stories, we would probably see some indication of how the idea of narrative entered into the story, how it was implemented, and the "problems" it faced and created. We know that before a program gets started it is suggested by some one, resisted by someone, approved by someone, funded, started, and evaluated. Cohen discusses an innovative program "The New Ideas Fund," which was started in order to ". . . encourage the development and testing of innovative ideas generated by public child welfare workers" (Cohen, 1999, p. 490). It was hoped that this could minimize the negative aspects of a large bureaucratic organization. He notes that this approach to organizational change is based on three design principles:

140

1. Worker participation in organizational improvement should be designed into the organizational structure and formally sanctioned.
2. Participation in organizational improvement should be built into the professional social worker's role and should be seen as part of the job.
3. Opportunities for individual and organizational learning should be designed and actively managed throughout the change process.

While these principles have guided QWL (Quality of Life) effort and the New Ideas Fund, their potency has been diminished by external events (e. g., a class action lawsuit that challenged the agency's practices and diverted attention), by continuing management-labor unrest and by fluctuations in top management support for the project. (Cohen 1999, p. 56)

There is obviously a story here that would help us understand how new programs are dealt with in agencies, and some steps that need to be taken. While we have stories about how practitioners became interested in the ideas of narrative (White, 1995a) we know less about how agencies accept or reject the idea of narrative practice.

Why this lack of attention to agency? The reason may very well be that many of the practitioners are in private practice or see themselves as autonomous practitioners who would function the way they do with or without an agency setting. The importance of the agency in narrative practice is highlighted in the work that Michael White did with the "Power to our Journeys" group (Bridgette, Sue, Mem, & Veronica, 1966). Following the development of the group, they went on to try to influence other organizations to modify their approaches and use the materials they had developed with White.

Most social work practice is carried out in an agency setting. While there are differences between public and private agencies, the function of the agency is the same, to offer a service on behalf of people (Addams, 1935; Richmond, 1917). The profession has consistently recognized its strong reliance on the social agency as the context for, and the shaper of practice.

The functionalist-oriented social work educators at the University of Pennsylvania, held that the agency function was a major factor in the helping process. Bertha Reynolds (1965) inherently understood the historic importance of the agency in social work as a contextual force and wrote, "For better or worse, the agency and its place in the community, its policies and questionings, influence profoundly all that (. . . the worker) personally may do" (1965, p. 205). She recognized the cogency of a democratic "social work" administrative climate for a profession involved in a struggle to integrate new scientific knowledge with its strong moral base. Influenced by the Freudian theory of the time she recognized the symbolic role of the administrator as the person who would be the role model and the catalyst for staff development, sensitive and intelligent practice, and close interactions with the community.

A narrative approach to administration promotes a participatory environment, of staff, of management, and of the client community. It can minimize the processes that prevent an agency from practicing in ways that provide the most competent use of staff and the promotion of the agency's mission. The agency becomes a living symbol for clients and staff as to the kinds of interactional processes that demonstrate the respectful treatment of persons.

Social work administration must always be "social work" administration. That is, while it shares common administrative management prerogatives related to goal attainment and common technologies, as well as basic organizational behavior theories, its intent, actions, and consequences are always related to the purposes, processes, and values of the profession. As William Schwartz (1974) noted,

> Every agency is an arena for the conversion of private troubles into public issues. The agency begins, in fact as an effort to provide a service that is of specific consequences both to society and to its individuals; each system is a special case of the individual-social encounter . . . the fact remains that the basic relationship between an institution and its people is symbiotic— each needs the other for his own survival . . . Each agency, on its part needs to justify its existence by serving the people for whom it was assigned. It is a form of social contract . . . (1974, p. 359)

The agency has a story that has shaped its behavior. Often the administrator is paramount in authoring the story, but the staff has an important part to play. Reynolds noted,

> It is true that many executives are arbitrary because they do not know how to work through and with other people, and it is also true, as we have said, that staff expect them to be, because staff have not learned how to carry their share of administrative responsibility . . . (1965, p. 322)

The staff is part of the agency narrative and influences the direction of the service. Whatever boundaries exist that separate administrative positions from staff positions, these boundaries are open when it concerns adequate service being provided to clients. It is important for staff to help the administrators do a good job, as it is for the administrators to ensure that the staff has the resources they need to be effective.

The task of incorporating a narrative practice orientation in carrying out administrative responsibilities is more complex than in working with an individual or even a group. The reason is that while the agency story has its own landscape and goals that must be authored over time, so do each of the staff members. This compounds the task of the administrator, not that they are therapists to the staff, but they are persons who have control over policies, processes, and attitudes that shape the climate or culture of the agency, and thus creates the context for a large part of the life of the staff. It is striking that in a democratic society, the largest part of the waking life of most working people in the United States is spent in a workplace where they have little, if anything, to say about their situation (Abels, 1973).

In addition, it would be unrealistic to discuss the matter of administration without accepting the reality that a great deal of power in a social agency, as in most organizations, resides in the hands of the administrator or the "administration." Whether we talk about administration as a group that is in charge of a project or organization, or administration as a process of running a project, there is no way not to accept the reality that someone or some group is "directing" something in which other people are involved. This seemingly conflicts with the notion that the worker is not the expert. Staff turns to and expects the administration to solve the problems in the agency just as clients expect the worker to solve the problems they face (Abels, 1977a).

Faced with this reality, we need to search for administrative practices that recognize the value of staff as persons, minimizes hierarchical power, and promotes democratic processes at all levels. The ideas of narrative administration then, ought to attempt not to privilege some staff over others, and yet accept that there are role differentials in which people have different skills, training, and experience that are necessary for the optimal operation of the project. Such an organization would also have to establish an equality of rights within the organization, and flatten the reward structure as well. Is it possible to have such organizations? Does our culture promote such organizational behavior? There are a few which come to mind; some have existed in the idea of communes, a few of which have been established and running for years. Lately there has been the celebration of equality in some entreprenurial start-up companies in the computer and e-mail business, but we are not aware of any large social agencies that have been able to function at such a high level.

We do know, however, that there have been organizations in the welfare arena such as settlement houses, which have tried to model that approach. The following is an excerpt from a settlement house director. Note that he refers to himself as the "head worker," and that residents was a term used in the early settlement days for the workers, some paid, some volunteer (Woods, 1970).

> As to the direction of the residents, there ought to be just enough authority in the head worker to make sure that unity and continuity are fairly kept up in the work of the settlement. It ought to be possible at any time to turn the whole force of the settlement down a single channel. But in dealing with the individual workers, I consider that it is essential to the plan of having educated persons doing intimate personal work, that the directions of the head worker should wholly take the form of suggestions, except in some rare instances, when his command or veto should be subject to appeal to the body of residents or to the managing council. It is not well even that the personality of one person should overshadow the rest, unless that person have much greater experience than they do. The general lines of action being assigned according to the inclinations of the residents, they ought to be expected to develop a great share of the invention and originality, which their own field of effort demands. The head worker ought to know everything that is being done by all the residents, and ought to be ready to offer suggestions and cautions whenever they seem to be needed. His suggestions may be especially frequent and pointed if he find any residents who are inclined to turn settlement work into a pastime. But, on the whole, it is indispensable to the scheme that every resident from the beginning should feel a possessive, creative interest in his own work; that he should feel not merely the cheerful glow of action, but that he should feel the lofty joy which the artist feels. Anything that hinders the entrance of such fine influence into the doing of the work will prevent it from being imparted as a result of the work. The life and soul of settlement work is the arm and magic that lingers about persons, with fetters off, and held only by a noble enthusiasm. (Woods, p. 23)

This example brings us very close to the philosophical approach of narrative. There is recognition that the "resident's" story is important. Orders and directions can stifle the creativity of the worker and that the work must come out of the ideas of the life of the group. Clearly, this administrator sees the importance of minimizing the hierarchy, and uses what would now be seen as participatory decision making. He recognizes the importance of the staff as a team and the agency as a community.

If the "administration" wants to empower its staff, it needs to take the same philosophical position that Pinderhughes (1995) suggests we take when we work to empower our clients: ". . . practitioners need to be knowledgeable about the dynamics of power and powerlessness and how these forces operate in human functioning. Moreover, practitioners must be able and willing to apply such knowledge to themselves as well as clients" (Pinderhughes, p. 133).

Power is not just in the hands of administration; staff has the responsibility of recognizing that they have the ability to shape the agency, and they must use their knowledge and skills to help administration use their power judiciously and on behalf of participatory practices, including the involvement of clients and various other systems in the community in order to help shape the direction of the agency.

Often the use of volunteers, particularly board members related to the community, has made such shared empowering possible. Profit sharing in corporations is a recent attempt to share income more equally among the workers and some of the initial computer and web companies have shared both power and finances, particularly as they start up. This has permitted other organizations to look at the potential of such hierarchically minimized organizations as possibilities. As the welfare area became a mammoth undertaking, most of the face-to-face, idealistic staff "chat" sessions evaporated. The metaphor of agency as a "family" or "community" was difficult to maintain in large highly bureaucratic structures. With the increase of privatization of social agency services, the intimate professional mission that staff felt in the past turns to their feeling alienated and like cogs in a wheel.

While Foucault (1980) has pointed out that power exists and can be changed at all levels, clearly in an agency most persons would agree that most of the power lies in the hands of the administrator and the board of directors. The way that administration is perceived and perceives its functions will influence the direction of the agency and the beliefs of the staff as to what degree their voices are heard.

The landscape of administration reveals a long historical process of change from an entirely authoritarian overseeing of the workers in the organization to an enlightened stance arising in part from research such as the Hawthorne studies, and in the 1970s and 1980s of the Japanese management style. Regardless of the historical rhetoric, the most influential shaping of management theory came out of the work of Frederick Taylor (1911) and scientific management. While the image is of him standing with a stopwatch to time and analyze separate movements of a particular job, his ability to systematize the workplace has had lasting repercussions. It is still a vital force in the management theory of the day.

The ideas of "span of control," of being responsible to only one supervisor, of the need for training and supervision, and the splitting of functions, are contributions he made which are still in use in modern management theory. Some lead to increased productivity without additional costs to the worker and in fact help make the work place safer, all in the name of increased production, of course. But many of the innovations tended to treat the worker as an object, a part of a machine that could be replaced. An example from his book *Scientific Management*, which served as a "bible" for many administrators, illustrates some of his philosophy and practice.

The task before us, then narrowed itself down to getting Schmidt to handle forty-seven tons of pig iron per day and making him glad to do it. This was done as follows: Schmidt was called out from among the gang of pig-iron handlers and talked to somewhat in this way:

"Schmidt, are you a high-priced man?" . . .

"Vell, I don't know vat you mean."

"Oh come now, you answer my questions. What I want to find out is whether you are a high-priced man or one of these cheap fellows here. What I want to find out is whether you want to earn $1.50 a day or whether you are satisfied with $1.15."

"Did I want $1.85 a day? Vot dot a high-priced man? Vell, yes, I was a high-priced man." . . .

"You see that car?"

"Yes."

"Well if you are a high-priced man, you will load that pig iron on that car tomorrow for $1.85. Now do wake up and answer my question. Tell me whether you are a high priced man or not." . . .

"Vell dot's all right. I could load dot pig iron on the car tomorrow for $1.85, and I get it every day, don't I?"

"Certainly you do—certainly you do."

"Vell den, I was a high-priced man."

"Now hold on, hold on, You know just as well as I do that a high-priced man has to do exactly as he is told from morning till night. You have seen this man here before, haven't you?"

"No, I never saw him."

"Well if you are a high-priced man, you will do exactly as this man tells you tomorrow, from morning till night. When he tells you to pick up a pig and walk, you pick it up and walk, and when he tells you to sit down and rest, you sit down. You do that right through the day. And what's more, no back talk. Now a high-priced man does just what he's told to do, and no back talk. Now you come on to work here tomorrow morning and I'll know before night whether you are really a high-priced man or not."

This seems to be rather rough talk. And indeed it would be if applied to an educated mechanic or even an intelligent laborer. With a man of the mentally sluggish type of Schmidt, it is appropriate and not unkind, since it is effective in fixing his attention on the high wages which he wants and away from what if it were called to his attention, he would probably consider impossibly hard work" (Taylor, pp. 57–60).

His book was translated into a number of languages, and went through numerous editions. It is important to reflect on Taylor's work in the context of the times. The idea of enlightened management and participatory workplaces were not yet on the scene. The idea of the manager of the department as boss was an important one. Workers were not given breaks, they were controlled by all kinds of rules, and there were few regulations about workers' rights or even safety. This was typified by the Triangle Shirt-waist fire. The fire doors were chained shut because the women would go out on the fire escape to have a smoke. Over a hundred women died in the fire. The authority of the boss was carried out by threat and by a simple "gaze" which indicated something was wrong. Foucault talks about the gaze as a mechanism of control; many of us have been subject to the look or frown that somehow signifies to us that we have not done right, by a parent, a teacher, and at times by a therapist. White mentions this as well, and also Jeremy Bentham's idea of the Panopticon, a prison in which the prisoners could be seen, but never knew when they were being watched. This, it was suggested would lead to them controlling their own behavior.

The insulting manner in which Taylor speaks to Schmidt sounds odd to us today, made even stranger by his writing it with his version of Schmidt's accent. It would certainly be politically incorrect to do so now. But there have been recent examples of minorities being ridiculed in corporate back rooms, and even in social agencies.

What is clear from this excerpt is that in the context of Taylor's times, the story of the agency was the only story which counted, and its plot needed to be carried out no matter what the cost to the persons in the organization. Regardless of the organization's goals, Schmidt had his own vision, and worked to re-author his own life. *Reflection: Have you come across people making fun of other people's accents? What kinds of jobs do recent immigrants get?*

While we do not intend to give a history of administrative and management theory at this juncture, it is important to note that the changes that have taken place, at least in many of the industrialized countries at this time, represent a move toward a more worker-centered administration. This might be a sign of enlightenment, or it might be related to the organizational research findings. These indicate that workers who are treated more respectfully and feel they have some say in the decisions that impact their lives tend to be more satisfied on the job. They remain on the job longer, may be more productive, and in some organizations, offer suggestions that helps the organization run more efficiently. One such example is the increased productively resulting from "quality circles" used widely in Japanese firms, although "invented" in the United States years before its use by Japanese management.

Professionals have always felt that their status in an organization differed from the role of the regular line worker. They have often held a dual loyalty, loyalty to the organization in which they were employed, and loyalty to their profession and its moral and ethical requirements. They have often counted on the power of their professional organizations to represent their interests. For example, the medical profession has never been interested in unionizing until recently when decisions about health care and their autonomy have been challenged by insurance companies. They have felt that in a professionally oriented setting they would have more authority than workers in a profit-oriented company in which there is some product or an assembly line. The medical profession, for example, felt it should be the power in a hospital. Professors believed similarly about their role in the University. The variation here differs, but there seems to be a demise of the professional role in decision making in such organizations. A major case in point is the medical profession, and their concern that medical decisions are being taken out of their hands.

Since the emergence of Health Maintenance Organizations (HMOs) and corporate-run social welfare services, some welfare institutions have tended to become more like large traditional profit-making corporations. The normative concept that the doctor should be the decision maker as to what services a patient should receive has been mitigated by business managers, insurance companies, and at times clerks who follow some prearranged list of what is permissible. This loss of decision-making power has created chagrin for the profession as well as the patients and is currently a major factor in the evolution of a national Patients' Bill of Rights.

While the battle is still one of control, it raises the question of who should have the control. Clearly, the code of ethics of the medical profession which puts the needs of the patients ahead of the need for profit would lead us to opt for the profession's control. We still must face the fact, however, that when any profession starts to monopolize a service, it may deter others from offering a service that might be better. One example was in the area of Psychiatry, which has always prevented and limited the types of service that nonmedical helpers could provide. While Freud believed that lay people should be able to offer psychiatric services, he was opposed in his thinking by the medical profession. Currently, efforts by psychologists to pass laws which would permit them to prescribe drugs under certain conditions is opposed by the medical profession. Efforts by nurses to increase their roles in the medical field, while initially opposed, has led to the evolution of the "nurse practitioner," a valuable resource in medical service, particularly in areas where medical doctors were scarce or nonexistent. Currently, there are states where the psychiatrist is trying to prevent licensing of social workers unless they work under the authority of the psychiatrist.

What we see is that power is at the heart of all organizational structures, with the power generally emanating from the top of the triangle, the "administration." Yet, efforts are made to minimize that power, particularly by professionals who at times see their work threatened by administrative decisions based on the need for the maintenance of the organization, its need for funds, and its efforts to reflect what the community might believe to be important such as "the agency should be run like a business." This creates a tension which at times interferes with the best possible service being made available to the clients.

The stories created by these tensions often become part of the culture and the history of the agency. These stories often determine the ability to attract the highest quality staff, funds, and at times clients. Where clients have a choice, they will go to the agencies that provide a competent and respectful workforce. Valence operates on workers too. When workers have a choice, they will seek employment in settings where they are given an opportunity to do the kind of work they like and which is challenging, and where staff are treated with respect.

In the portions of this chapter which follow we will examine some of the efforts of major organizations to incorporate normative practice approaches in the operating principles of their organization and in their administrative practice.

We would like to start first with some of the thoughts that the authors have had over the years as to kinds of administrative practices in the social services that would best serve the goals of our profession. The idea is that social justice as a goal for our clients should be as important a goal for the agency administrator to consider in his/her approach to staff and board. In essence, what was a sound vision for the clients was equally sound for work with staff.

In *Administration in the Human Services: A Synergistic Systems Approach* (Abels & Murphy, 1981), Abels introduced what he believed was an approach to administration which led to more of an interactional and relational form of administration which would benefit the staff, the clients, and the agency. It was referred to as a "normative" model, normative in the sense of "what ought to be" if we were going to provide the kind of service that meets the vision of our profession. It suggested that management in social work had similarities with management in other fields but also differed in style, purpose, and ways of assessing success. It also suggested that staff in a social agency had a different voice than in many other types of organizations. It also had a major role to play in sharing knowledge freely with the community it serves, a role which many for-profit organizations might play, but hardly ever do carry out. A brief summary of its major points will help the reader see its verisimilitude with a number of the principles inherent in the narrative approach, and reflect social work's values as well.

We believe that some of the principles outlined below reflect an organizational approach that would promote the success of narrative practice, and would itself use such processes in working with staff.

1. All people should be treated with respect and dignity.
2. The results of our actions should lead to "just consequences."
3. Worker actions should lead to increased freedom for the clients.
4. Worker actions should be state-of-the-art.
5. Staff should be treated with the same respect and dignity as the clients.
6. Staff should participate in the decision making in the agency.
7. An agency is a group of persons working together for the benefit of the clients.

A major effort to examine how the narrative approach might be used in organizational change was carried out by Carl Rhodes (1996). Rhodes did a qualitative research study to see how the benefits of a narrative approach might be incorporated into work with organizations. His emphasis, however, was primarily on how the telling of stories influences change in the organization. Rhodes did not carry his findings a step further to show how the stories might be re-authored. This is a universal problem, mitigated by the separation of research from practice in many fields.

ADMINISTRATIVE CONTROL:
SENSE MAKING AND ABUSES

As mentioned previously, White makes a point of the work of Jeremy Bentham and the Panopticon, which was a design aimed at developing a prison system in which the inmates would be trained in a sense to control their own behavior. This was done by setting up the prison in such a way that a guard sitting in a central location could see in the cells by the way they were arranged and lit. The prisoners could not know if they were being observed or not. This put them in a position of being on their best behavior because they never knew when someone would be watching them (McKinlay & Starkey, 1997). The television show OZ is a graphic drama depicting life in such a modern prison.

While this may make sense for convicts, does the same philosophy make sense in an organization? A headline in the *New York Times* read "TheWeb; New Ticket to a Pink Slip; On the job, the Boss Can Watch Your every Online Move, and You Have Few Defenses" (Guernsey, 1999). The article begins:

> One time early in October, forty employees of the Xerox corporation working in locations across the United States received unwelcome news: They had been caught in the act of surfing to forbidden Web sites, nabbed not by managers or fellow employees but by software designed to monitor their online indiscretions. The software recorded every web site they had visited (many of which it turned out were related to shopping or pornography) and every minute they spent at those sites.

This is just the most recent example of attempts to control worker behavior. There are a few limitations on what can be controlled. For example, the employer cannot go into your personal desk drawer if it is locked, and listen in on private phone calls unless you have been previously told that this will occur. In a letter to the editor, a reader commented that any organization that has such regulations should also not permit their workers to think about the organization during their time off the job. The writer pointed out how much people often think about ways to solve some agency problem while they are off the job, while driving for example (*New York Times*, Dec. 23, 1999).

NARRATIVE APPROACHES TO ADMINISTRATION

In an effort to examine the contribution that Narrative Therapy might make in the promoting of organizational change, Barry asks, "How might narrativist writings, which tend to take a nonutilitarian, postmodernist slant, be used to inform organizational change, which is often enacted in distinctly utilitarian and modernist ways?" He answers that some steps in that direction already exist in agencies that take the view "client knows best," noting that the action research schools have always taken that view (Barry, 1997, p. 32). Considering the fact that Narrative Therapy has shown it works with individuals, couples, and families, he is intrigued by the possibility of its use for organizational change. He points out how often the metaphor of family is used by the organization, class, paternalistic systems, and multigenerational cultures. Issues of identity, survival, power, and social positioning are issues found in all organizations.

As a consultant to a health agency, he decided to attempt to work with the agency using the narrative philosophy and techniques. It was difficult to avoid his old framework, developing a strategy, suggesting better accounting or a gainshare program. Instead, he started to listen to the internalizing conversations of the two organizational people he was consulting with. Two things began to emerge—administrative competence and overwork.

He composed a letter which he sent them in which he used the externalized problems as a source of raising their awareness. "For now, your collective story seems to resolve around two characters. Overwork and Administrative Angst." Later he adds, "We also wonder if you've started bringing the rest of the staff into this picture . . . what is their relationship to Administrative Angst and Overwork? How might they tell their story?" He closes with the following, "Have others noticed the changes you've started to make? What are your thoughts about this?" (p. 32)

While he was doing this, he had a number of doubts as to whether it would be successful, but the organization increased its productivity; people reported doing less work and being more satisfied, They . . . "said the narrative work had fundamentally changed their practice, it seemed too good to be true. Could these few 'artful' stories help so much? Maybe this was all some enormous placebo effect, some self-fulfilling prophecy." In conclusion, he summarizes some of his observations,

> I was struck by how piecemeal organizational stories are, particularly problem saturated ones. . . . I have also became aware that this approach has little to do with solving problems (at least not directly); rather it is about changing the relationship people have with their problems.

He concludes that his experiment led him to believe that narrative can work in organizations, particularly with small groups, and he suggests ways this might be accomplished. He was also impressed with the success of the letters, and pointed out how large organizations might use this technique with people out of everyday touch with the agency. His article leaves many questions unanswered but would lead the reader to think that its use is very possible. This was a small organization and the two partners in the business were willing to give this new approach a try. This might give us a clue to believe that it may work best in a smaller agency, and not a large welfare department. However, it is our experience that even in larger organizations individual workers can use narrative if the administration is not bound to a particular approach to helping.

INITIATING NARRATIVE IN THE AGENCY

In order to be most effective in applying the narrative approach as a model of help within the social agency, there must be some consensus among the staff that this is an approach worthy of being implemented. Unless the agency is starting from scratch, some of the workers are going to have privileged approaches which they believe are important for them to use. It would be important to introduce the ideas of postmodernism, with some reading and possibly a speaker, not to push narrative but rather to look at why the times are calling for new ways of appraising practice. It might then make sense to examine narrative practice, either by readings, a speaker, or both.

Is it necessary for all workers to move into narrative? Of course not. To force such an effort would be violating some of the basic principles not only of narrative, but also the ethical imperatives of our profession. But it would be important for the staff to know about narrative prior to their having to make some decision regarding its use in the agency. It might suffice to obtain agreement from one person to initiate it with clients and then to have staffings on a regular basis to examine just what the process looks like. Of course if the person introducing the idea was the person who undertook the task of the narrative experiment it might enable others not to feel that someone had to volunteer. It is not necessary that the idea to try narrative come from the executive, but it would certainly be important for the person to discuss it with the executive prior to any open meetings on the subject. The administration's support would be very important or at least administrative neutrality if not support. Opposition

from the administrator would be the death knell of an effort to incorporate narrative in the range of helping offered within the agency.

In addressing how the New Ideas Fund might be introduced into
other agencies, Cohen (1999) warns that several factors are essential:

> First, there must be an individual or small group who will be the driving
> force. This can be initially an insider or an outsider . . . Second, there
> needs to be some role that has been played by the Steering Committee.
> Third, there needs to be some commitment of resources, either internal,
> external, or both. Finally and most importantly, top management has to
> show strong support for the project, but be willing to sit back and allow it
> to unfold, recognizing that the forces unleashed may alter the organiza-
> tion. (p. 58)

While the authors agree with Cohen's ideas, it may be very difficult for
administration to sit back if the changes are going to be seen as threatening to them, and these need to be dealt with as they evolve.

Harlene Anderson (1997) sees the organization as,

> . . . yet another purposeful social system that has formed around a particu-
> lar value preference. Such systems share the complexities of systems that
> we meet in therapy and in teaching. . . .
>   Like therapy and teaching, organizational consultation involves con-
> necting, collaborating and constructing . . . dialogue remains the essence
> of the consultation process . . . I want to provide a conversational space
> and facilitate a conversational process in which the client(s) can engage in
> dialogue with himself or herself . . . Such collaborative inquiry moves
> from the top-down elite problem solving process to a shared process that
> involves multiple problem solvers. . . . (p. 259)

The use of small discussion groups and then large groups to reflect
together was part of her consultation process. She ends the process with
mutual reflections by the participants and the worker. She also notes the
importance of recording the sessions and the process as these become
important ways of reviewing and reflecting on what happened, and making it available to everyone.

The workers in private practice can pretty much decide for themselves
whether or not they want to initiate narrative practice in their work. The
worker in the agency, whether the administrator or a line staff person, has
a more complicated task. There are often resistances to change, and both
Kurt Lewin and R. Lippit have dealt with ways in which resistance to

change may be accommodated in the agency without creating major problems for the staff (Lewin, 1958; Lippit, Watson, & Westly, 1958). In addition, a group which called itself "Synetics" worked on extremely creative approaches to change.

Alex Gitterman (Gitterman & Shulman, 1994), in a very practical, illustrative article, discusses ways in which new programs can be developed in agencies. He notes,

> Complex agencies, characterized by a large number of professional disciplines have been found to be more responsive to programmatic innovation. The diversity and advanced training create a greater openness to new ideas, methods, and technologies and therefore offer the worker a certain degree of organizational maneuverability. At the same time, the actual program implementation requires complex coordination with numerous turf-conscious disciplines . . . (Gitterman, p. 62)

There are often resistances to new programs. The reasons are many including funds, time, entrenched programs, and allegiance to certain models. William Schwartz (1961), who was successful in moving us into new areas of social work practice, noted the difficulties of introducing new practice perspectives,

> . . . those who have been schooled in social group work (social work) have a rich store of experience to contribute. The task is, of course, rendered doubly difficult by the fact that any worker who attempts it must break the bonds of his/her own training since they (have) been reared in ancient fallacies. (Schwartz, 1961, p. 150)

The agency administrator is in a good position to initiate change within the organization. The administrator, however, must be cognizant that the consequences of his/her actions needs to lead to "good" outcomes. We suggest that there are two important factors that need to be considered in such actions. The first is that the agency needs to introduce practice that is effective, and second, that the actions need to be introduced in a democratic, participatory manner. An important principle to consider is that just as the client is their own best consultant, the staff that will need to work with the new program are the best consultants as to what they need to know in order to do a good job.

When the staff have not been helped to work together the results often reflect poor service to the clients. At times the lack of training can have catastrophic results. One example of this was the death of fire jumpers due to a lack of trust in their leader and poor training as a team as described in Weick's brilliant article (1993) on sensemaking. The narrative he presents about the incident helps us understand the importance of creative administrative leadership. His comparisons with the way airline teams are trained provides a valuable illustration of participatory decision making.

America Bracho (2000) discusses a number of programs developed by the Latino community dealing with health and community building showing the importance of involving the community in the administration of programs. This is vital if the community is to feel the program is theirs.

10

Multicultural Narrative Practice

They approach me in a half-hesitant sort of way, eye me curiously or compassionately, and then, instead of saying directly, How does it feel to be a problem? They say, I know an excellent colored man in town, or, I fought at Mechanicsville; or Do not these Southern outrages make your blood boil? At these I smile, or am interested, or reduce the boiling to a simmer, as the occasion may require. To the real question, How does it feel to be a problem? I answer seldom a word.

(W.E.B. DuBois, *The Souls of Black Folk*)

Helen Perlman once said, "life . . . in itself is a problem solving process" (Perlman, 1957, p. 53). Does DuBois suggest that for him in addition to solving the usual life problems, he must deal with the problem of people seeing him as a problem? Are people really problems? Is the story of his experience a narrative of the African-American experience as well? Could Perlman's statement be altered to read: "life is a series of stories we are told and tell ourselves about others and ourselves?" Do some of these stories help us solve problems, or do some cause additional problems for us? Do some stories denigrate us, do some uplift us, do some suggest we are problems? Where do these stories come from? How are problem stories created? Who in the world decides what a problem is, and who decides that a whole group of people are problems? Who decides who the problem solvers should be?

By now we have examined these questions, and we know some of the answers. But many questions remain. Can the social work profession really deal with the catastrophic social problem that DuBois so ably personalized? In 1940, Myrdal wrote a book called *The American Dilemma*.

Racism and prejudice was the "dilemma." The Civil Rights Commission reporting on the riots presented the same dilemma to us. We have been a racist society and we still are. Many people see certain groups as problems, be they minorities, gays and lesbians, Jews, or Muslims (Ellison, 1989; Friedman, 1973; Karenga, 1998; Reynolds, 1931). While strides have been made to "overcome," a look at the daily news will remind of us the hate crimes, civil rights abuses, and stigma that some people in our society are subject to.

Who is the enemy? Who are the people who make statements such as, "they are simply lazy, immoral and ignorant." "All they want to do is have babies, watch television, and stick us with the bill." "They are a threat to what is good about this country." "They are destroying family values." Verbal attacks such as these are just the tip of the iceberg because in many cases violence and even death are companions to these statements. Welfare developments such as The Personal Responsibility and Work Opportunity Reconciliation Act only serve to intensify the problems that the poor face in our country. Privatization of services, and the widening gap between the wealthy and the poor and middle classes has intensified a callousness for the oppressed (Piven & Cloward, 1971).

What we see and hear is in large part a measure of perception in a multicultural society that is increasingly characterized by painful and often paralyzing inequities. Some have suggested that selective perception is necessary to avoid seeing the pain and suffering of others. We have clearly seen this with the homeless. Instead of seeing them, we have become impervious to their existence by redefining their reality. "They could find jobs if they wanted to." "They could find housing if they wanted to," even though we know that the cost of housing is out of their reach. Even though we know that many of the homeless are emotionally unable to work.

Seeing and hearing those who are devalued in our society has become the domain of the social work profession. We have heard the horror stories of living life close to the bone day after day. Is anyone else listening?

WHOSE VOICES WILL BE HEARD?

There are a number of persons whose voices are rarely heard. These are often members of minority groups, the poor, even certain professions such as social work (Abels & Oliver, 1997; Liebow, 1993; Pear, 2000). Having a "voice" has become a metaphor related to civil rights, equality, resistance, liberation, and power. Perhaps the most clarion call for their voice being heard has come from women, exemplified by books such as *In a Different Voice* by Carol Gilligan (1982). Being heard seems to be the major way a group is recognized, not to downplay being seen, as in Ralph Ellison's *Invisible Man* (1989), but the voice seems to be the dominant way of acknowledgment of one's existence. Even a person seen is usually acknowledged by a verbal message. "Hello, how are you?"

To the degree that you have power, you have a voice. Who speaks for those whose voices are ignored (Niebuhr, 1999)? A difficult question to ask, since as social workers we have been alerted to the pitfalls of trying to represent the ideas of others, or to speak on their behalf, even for the best of reasons. Perhaps we can say that we speak for social justice, and not for any one group (Lee, 1994; Saleebey 1992, 1994). It has always been social work's mandate to represent the best needs of the poor and oppressed in our society. That is our profession's heroic contract. If not the poor, then us. If not the oppressed, then us. If not us, then who (Schwartz, 1974)?

People want their voices heard. They want the world to know about their struggles, their attempts to overcome, their oppression, their ignored needs, and their bravery as they survive in the face of callous disregard. We become the ones who they are counting on to tell their story. Eliot Liebow's book, *Tell them Who I Am: The Lives of Homeless Women* (1993), is just such a current narrative. Those are the stories of brave people whose daily struggle make them heroes, keeping their families and lives together in the face of a voiceproof society (Abels, 1971; Gitterman & Shulman, 1994).

Bridgitte and others discuss their attempts to gain power over their lives (Bridgitte, Sue, Mem, & Veronica, 1996):

> We would like to introduce ourselves as members of the Power to Our Journeys group based in Dulwich Centre in Adelaide, Australia. We would like you to know that all of us have been recipients of mainstream psychiatric services for varying lengths of time, have been subject to various treatments, and have all been assigned various diagnoses over this time. The people who have treated us have mostly settled on the diagnosis of schizophrenia. . . .
>
> Over the many years of our different connections with psychiatric services, we have found little opportunity to speak openly of our day-to-day experiences of the voices and visions that have been so troublesome to us, or, for that matter, the voices and visions that have been helpful to our lives. We have been silenced time and again by many psychiatric professionals who have constantly refused to acknowledge our experiences of these voices and visions. (p. 11)

They go on to discuss the group they started with the help of Michael White and their attempts to influence the mental health system.

THE LANDSCAPE OF CULTURE

Where do some of the stories that shape our lives come from? Most are learned at an early age from the family, from the schools, and from religious institutions we may have attended in our youth. All of these, however, are greatly influenced by the cultures which served as a context for our experiences in the past and which are relevant to our present lives. This is particularly cogent for those who may have moved from the country of their childhood to a new country, or for a person whose cultural values differ from those of the culture which dominates his/her ecosystem (Green, 1995; Rasheed & Rasheed, 1999; Weaver, 1999). There are many areas of dispute as to the role of culture. The nature-nurture argument is just one. Is there such a thing as the culture of poverty, or a culture of youth, or of gays, or of the aged? But there is general agreement that cultural factors are a strong influence on the world view of persons both as individuals or as a group and society.

Social workers' understanding of cultural influence has come primarily from the fields of anthropology and sociology. Those disciplines tend to define culture as:

> . . . the way of life of a particular society or group of people, including patterns of thought, beliefs, behavior, customs, traditions, rituals, dress, and language, as well as art, music, and literature. The primary use of the term is in the social sciences where it refers to the whole way of life both material and spiritual of a particular society. (Brockhampton, 1994, p. 130)

The *Blackwell Dictionary of Sociology* (Johnson, 1995) gives us a definition which offers another perspective to the idea of culture. It notes that, "culture is the accumulated store of symbols, ideas and material products associated with a social system, whether it be an entire society or a family" (p. 68).

These groups, whether or not they are nationally oriented, religiously similar, age-related, or of the same gender or ethnicity, are often privileged to have similar stories that reflect their culture, the teachings, and the environmental forces in the context of their development, or the forces influencing them in their current environment. Many women from different cultural backgrounds can tell you the story of the "glass ceilings" which they encountered regardless of their capabilities. Gays and lesbians, no matter what their religion, can relate stories of rejection by their congregations and discrimination in the armed forces. Handicapped persons, no matter what their gender, can tell similar stories of the lack of access to buildings and positions because of certain beliefs about them. The stories of most minorities share some plots related to being seen as less desirable than the mainstream citizen and being treated in a discriminatory fashion. The collection and interning of the American-Japanese in the United States during World War II is a case in point.

These are harsh and cruel stories, stories of oppression and neglect. Under certain conditions, the victims come to accept the stories they live as the truth. In many places women have accepted the "truth" of male superiority. At one time, homosexuals accepted others' views that they were "sick." So did many of the helping professionals, and homosexuals were listed as being so in the DSM, the clinical bible put out by the American Psychiatric Association, and used to identify certain behaviors as mental illness. Under pressure from various groups, the association by a narrow majority removed it from the DSM in the most recent volume (Volume IV).

In some instances, these are the stories that have led to the expansion of our profession into new areas of service, and promoted the growth of social work and motivated some persons to enter the field. The sense of injustice has always been an important motivator in our profession (Pumphrey & Pumphey, 1956; Sampson, 1999).

Holland and Kilpatrick (1993) have pointed out how these stories can be used to help students learn more about multicultural practice. Others have seen this as an area in which our practice has been less than perfect (Rasheed & Rasheed, 1999; Weaver, 1999).

In recent years, attention to multiculturalism has become an imperative in order for schools of social work to obtain accreditation. It is the authors' belief that our profession has been in the forefront of work for multicultural equality, often at a major risk to its survival either from political attacks or limitation of funds. In New York City funds meant for housing persons with AIDS were taken out of the hands of the mayor by the federal government because he was accused of using them as a political club against an organization that was critical of some of his actions. Representing the views of minorities, the poor, and the disenfranchised often means opposing the power structures and the established means of dealing with social problems. One of President Nixon's major aides warned social workers to get honest jobs. In an interview in *Reflections,*

Mitchel Ginsberg, who was the director of welfare for New York City, reports on that remark. The interviewer, Josua Miller asks, "Nixon disliked social workers, didn't he?" Ginsberg replied,

> Yes he did. But I have to say this about him, once when I met him and shook his hand, he said, "you have a tougher job than I have." But he disliked social workers and almost everybody else. I think one of my better quotes that ran in the *Wall Street Journal* on the front page, was [after] Haldeman had said, when Nixon got his welfare plan, there wouldn't be any jobs for social workers and they would have to go out and earn an honest living. I was President of NASW, and the *Journal*, among others, asked me for a quote or a comment and I said, "how would he know what an honest living is." (Miller, 1995, p. 58)

At times, our profession has pressed the fact that there are people who benefit from the social problems—for example, the availability of the cheap labor provided by immigrants and undocumented aliens. Some of these forces benefit by the existence of minimally helpful welfare programs. More recently we have started to support efforts opposing the insurance companies' influence over medical decisions in HMOs. The narrative therapists have openly attempted to deal with the oppression of the Australian Aborigines, a group that has faced genocide and a loss of their cultural identity. In the 2000 Olympics held in Australia there was a confrontation as to whether the Aborigines could fly their own flag at the ceremonies alongside the Australian flag.

THE MYSTIQUE OF MULTICULTURAL COMPETENCE

In its simplest, most pragmatic terms, multiculturalism refers to the recognition of the diversity of lifestyles, cultures, and backgrounds that make up the "body" of people who we work with in our profession. While in dictionary terms the culture may refer to a group with a particular language, lifestyle, artifacts, values, and so forth, we will take the broader view and accept the fact that there are certain preferences that may accompany gender, age, and economic lifestyles. For example, a certain style of dress, belief, acting, talking, while only partially different from the mainstream society, has evolved for whatever reasons as "different." While they may change within a decade or even a few generations they do form a recognizable pattern of behavior for that system.

These may be unfamiliar cultural artifacts to the worker. The worker cannot be an expert on all of these differences. It is not just language, speaking Spanish, for example, which may still require an interpreter to understand the current language of the teenage gang. It does not make a worker more familiar with their musical tastes or the importance of the gang to the members. Speaking Yiddish does not help one understand the "underground" culture of the Russian Jewish immigrant, their fear of authority or their desire for freedom. It is important, however, to understand how the cultural stories of the past are important connections for the client in the present (Rosenzweig & Thelen, 1998). J. D. Hamlet discusses the African-American sermon as a narrative (Hamlet, 1994).

We believe that a worker can never really understand any other person, regardless of the degree of verisimilitude with their own culture. The proof of this might be to ask, do you really understand yourself? Could your explain all of the motivations for your own actions? How then, can we claim to understand other cultures? The best we can do is to try to be aware of our own biases, our own shortcomings, and the importance of including the client in helping us to understand them and what they want us to do. This is a basic ingredient in the narrative approach, and has always been an important value in social work as well. Its importance was diminished as we sought models of helping that fed on the public's desire to find a quick fix to problems. We found ourselves seeking models that would strategize, instruct, impose, and demand certain actions from the client. While our hearts might have been in the right place, subject to pressures that negated our first principles, we succumbed. Like other professions, we would follow the bandwagon. Double-bind, strategic therapy, behavior modification, and paradoxical therapy all have had turns and been rejected or lost some of their influence. What we have found is that in most cases it made very little difference what model was used. Results were most often dependent on the nature of the relationship with the client, something that has always been a basic concept in social work, and is paramount in narrative practice.

For years the profession has been accused of leaving work with the poor and minorities to the public social services such as welfare departments and child welfare. Whether or not that is true is questionable as there are numerous accounts of workers in inner cities working with minorities, active both in individual counseling and in organizational and social change. There is no doubt, however, that until the war on poverty, the major efforts in that direction was usually carried out in the settlement houses, either by group workers or community organizers. The legislation

aimed at reducing poverty modified the profession somewhat and counseling became less prevalent for about a decade, only to emerge strongly
again with the growth of private practice. One catalyst for this re-growth
was the emergence of insurance-supported mental health services.

The question of the ability to work with people of a different background (other than whites or the middle class), has always been a major
concern in our profession (Reynolds, 1965) and has appeared in text-
books since the 1970s and 1980s (Devore & Schlesinger, 1987; Green,
1982). Following the civil rights movement of the 1970s there emerged a
major press by African-American and Latino/a social workers that the
profession become more active in social action and sensitive to minority
issues. For example, some suggested that the Genogram, a familiar tool in
the helping profession, might not be appropriate for African-American
families. Others suggest that Anglo social workers might not understand
minority families. There is a growing literature related to these ideas, some
of it suggesting that mainstream social workers cannot work with minorities,
and that such groups should have their own agencies (De Anda, 1977).

Weaver (1999) states that, "In part, striving for cultural competence is
a recognition of the profession's ethnocentric foundation" (p. 217). This,
she suggests, is because social work's historical roots were in England,
and that Eurocentric values have been propagated as universal and rigid-
ly imposed on clients. This view seems to ignore that there were significant contributions made by minority groups. It ignores as well, the battles
around the social security act in which many leaders fought provisions
seen as European and un-American. The problem of ethnocentrism,
while not limited to whites, has been an area of concern to social workers
and has been addressed in our profession for years. In general, the beliefs
about the need for social work to become more aware of cultural differences can be summed up by this statement by Kenneth Chau (1991),

> Although social work is committed to the well being of vulnerable and
> oppressed groups, the sociocultural reality of ethnic minority individuals has
> not been acknowledged by mental health professionals. Nor have the stress
> and strains of cultural differences or conflicts borne out of belonging to two
> cultures been fully recognized in the services provided to minorities. Despite
> increased acknowledgement of cultural variations in behavior, ethnic minori-
> ties continue to be assessed and treated according to the single definition of
> "normal" behavior of the mainstream of society. (Chau, p. 251, 1991)

During this period a number of studies were carried out by the Council
on Social Work Education on ethnicity and efforts to become aware of
the problems facing the minority in the helping situation.

In addition there was a major effort to recruit minorities into the field. While this has proven successful there still remains the problem of cross-cultural practice. Can someone of their own background better serve clients? Are the workers sensitive enough to the needs of a particular group? While these appear to be new concerns, the problem existed in religious settings before it became an ethnic or racial concern.

For example, from its inception the Jewish Family Services was established to serve the welfare needs of the Jewish community. At that time it was funded mainly through contributions from the Jewish community through various funding agencies such as the Jewish Federation. As part of their orientation they held the belief that the workers in direct service to the Jewish client should be Jewish, and with rare exceptions this remained the norm for many years. Over time the strict regulation began to be modified as the evidence that service by non-Jewish workers did not diminish the ability of the client to accept help and to respond positively to the experience. A shortage of staff may have added to the increased need to expand their services. The levels of practice and the results were comparable with what had been seen as a particularly religious need. While the non-Jewish workers were not aware of all the rituals, beliefs, and cultural artifacts of Jewish life, the capable worker was not at a disadvantage as ongoing training and supervision was available. Workers feeling a commitment to their clients will learn all they can that may be useful, and the idea that learning never ends makes the use of supervision in social work an acceptable and often a sought-after part of the practice experience.

We must, however, be particularly aware that there are conservative groups in all religious denominations that will hold values that restrict the use of some of the services that an agency might wish to offer, or even refuse to use an agency that differs from their views. Family planning is such an area of service; being open on the Sabbath is another; food and dress options also are sensitive issues. These are important considerations for both the agency and individual workers to consider.

MULTICULTURAL PRACTICE

Starting in the late 1960s increased efforts were undertaken to extend the knowledge workers have about the difference in the backgrounds and beliefs of clients whose culture might differ from that of the worker; in essence, to make the worker more culturally sensitive. While the catalyst was the ethnicity/racial issue, gender sensitivity was stressed as well.

Women spoke in a different voice. Changes in the approach to helping went along with the efforts to respond to this need for cultural understanding and texts began to appear in social work which reflected this move.

The theory of the "dual perspective" stressed the impact of both the person's cultural heritage and the surrounding culture, and how often different value orientations create personal stress, and how these differences need to be integrated in order to survive. The external culture, labeled at times as the "dominant," "mainstream," or even "Anglo" culture, was the culture that imposed its norms on the minority. (Note: certain words are "cue words" for minorities—"oppressed," "inner city," "New Yorkish").

Efforts were made to help people understand and value their own culture, and not to privilege the dominant culture. Postmodernists began to address the concepts of Eurocentricism and Afrocentricism, often leading to strong disagreements as to the reality of historic cultural claims as well as recognizing the importance of historic connections (Lefkowitz, 1996).

Helping approaches have not been able to adapt as easily as they would like. Given the alternative of providing a match between worker and client based on ethnicity, religion, gender, disability, and so on, presents an impossible situation and might reflect the absurdity of attempting such a match in an agency with limited resources and/or a cadre of workers without the training to follow through.

A review of the literature during the past few years indicates very little evidence that such efforts have been attempted on a large scale, and where attempted they have not been evaluated on a comparative basis. They have not yet demonstrated more than that people feel most comfortable with workers who are more like themselves. This has not transferred into effectiveness (Abels, 1997a). The one exception seems to be in the area of sexual abuse and rape of women, where women overwhelmingly prefer a female worker. In addition, literature reviews indicates that practice proposals offer little clues other than that the worker needs to be sensitive to the background culture of the client. As a practice innovation this offers no new direction.

NARRATIVE'S NATURAL CULTURAL RELEVANCE

Narrative practice presents a built in response to the call for culturally relevant practice. Recall its roots—many of the problems that all people face are created by social forces, perhaps unintentionally, but practically, to maintain power in the hands of those who can frame the political agendas.

Narrative practice not only takes into consideration the background of the person, but also helps them see how their culture and the external forces are paramount in the creation of the situation in which they find themselves. In addition, it is an approach that comes closest to mediating the status differential between worker and client. This is particularly important when there are cultural, ethnic, gender, and/or class differences between the clients and the worker, and/or when history suggests that one had also treated the other as inferior. This sets up a natural screen through which the client group assesses the helper. Can that person be trusted, or are there risks to confiding in that person? Will what is told be used against them? Is the helper on their side or an enemy who is ready to belittle them at a moment's notice? Narrative comes closest to helping the worker and the client team up, regardless of the nature of the backgrounds of either.

There are a number of factors supporting diversity in the narrative metaphor:

1. The idea that the client is their own best consultant permits the worker the freedom to call on anyone the client feels might help the worker understand the nature of the situation they present to him/her. If there is a language problem, then the client can bring someone to translate. If there is a gender issue, the client can bring a friend. Is there an age concern? The teenager can bring someone to keep them company during the interview, the aged person a partner. There is a freedom of constancy which fortifies the idea that the worker is really interested in helping the person, on their terms as much as "makes sense" to both parties.

2. Then there is the idea that the worker is not an expert. Admitting that the worker could use help in understanding the needs of the client holds to the narrative's opinion that they should not be seen as experts. That there are other views perhaps just as valuable as to what the client might need. When others are asked to participate in the helping situation, it not only acts as a mutual aid support, but also serves to offer other dialogues with the client about directions to be taken. Often, then, the views of the helper are discussed, reinforced, or seen as not helpful; to be brought back to the worker with questions and enlightened concern. There is an effort to minimize a judgmental approach by those augmented helpers. The training of the reflective team is an example of such an effort.

3. The worker "knows nothing" about the meaning of the experience to the client. The admission in some way by the worker that it is impossible

for them to understand the meaning of the experience creates the possibility of the client helping by interpreting, reminiscing, and working harder to mutually understand each other's tasks in the conversation. This admission goes beyond the worker not being an expert, but helps the client accept what they already know. "That nobody knows the trouble I've seen," no matter how the person explains that they understand, no matter how empathetic, the minority person knows that the worker of a different cultural background cannot really understand, feel for, or embrace their own history. There is a truth to this that cannot be talked away.

4. Then there is the idea that the person is not the problem. After constantly being told there is something wrong with you, a worker telling you that the problem has external causes and is out there, something which you already know to be true from your own lived experiences, is self-actualizing. We have discussed the power of externalizing before and need not repeat it other than to remind ourselves that this is extremely important for minorities who have generally been the groups oppressed by that external power structure.

We have seen countless references to self-hatred or feelings of worthlessness, to negating of their own culture, their own color, their own sex, and even their own bodies because of the rhetoric of the media and those with unbridled power. "Black is Beautiful" was a partial response to young African-American children selecting white dolls over black ones when given a choice, as well as other demeaning references to a particular group.

5. Telling their story, their way. The person is not presenting a problem; they are relating their story, the good parts and the bad, and are in a position of relating the positive parts of the stories. This can be extremely important. While being a slave is a position of utmost degradation, being able to relate the struggles and the powers of the persons who overcame that horror is a testament to their own worth. An example is the Jewish Passover tradition, which starts with the phrase "Once we were slaves in Egypt." It was something to be angry about, horrified about, but not to be ashamed of, something to be reminded of as proof of ability to survive, of leadership, and as a reminder to fight against oppression and for social justice.

6. The Reflecting Team offers different cultural, age, or gender views of what the client is going through and the actions they have taken. They are helpful to the person's seeing other views but also in getting support from people who may be familiar with the client's cultural milieu.

THE CONSTRUCTION OF THE POWERFUL

White has pointed out that "The culture of therapy is not exempt from the structures and ideologies of dominant culture," nor is it exempt from the influences of gender, race, class, age, ethnicity, and sexual preferences. A worker who understands this, and incorporates it into his/her practice and worldview, is more able to be tuned into the client's need to know that this worker will understand. Assuming a respectful willingness to listen and learn stance from the start of the session is one way of attempting to get across to the client this openness to the puzzle of the client, and the dedication of the worker to meet the client on their terms.

Beginning the sessions with lengthy forms to be filled out, with continuing questions about regulations as to the number of sessions that will be permitted, the need to be on time, the threat of being dropped from the client category if more than two sessions are missed, is oppressive. While these may be important to the agency, such a beginning usually puts the client in a position reminiscent of their powerlessness.

When the voice of the worker sounds like a parent, a boss, or even perhaps a "master," the client, particularly a minority client, is cast into a fight-or-flight stance. A client's resistance to an authoritarian worker may be an automatic move for survival, which might in this case be good or bad. To reject endless questions with a demand for "real help" may be utterance of the survival instinct that has kept the client going until now. Creating threatening contextual settings for helping does not make for the kind of relationship with the client that facilitates their working to re-author their lives. Their energy goes into self-preservation.

Certainly, accountability requires some information about the client, perhaps to ascertain eligibility, evaluate success, or to secure funding. Whatever the reason, the voices of authority are at play unless the client understands the necessity for some of the questioning, and unless questions are kept at a minimum and perceived as relevant by the client, they may do more harm than good. If the agency rules or worker style start to be important factors leading to a client feeling subjugated, then helping may be impossible. One might hold as a standard, what is the least amount of personal information I need to obtain prior to the conclusion of this first meeting in order to start the helping process.

Those in private practice certainly have the freedom to limit the number of questions that need to be asked in order to complete the necessary forms. Whether private practice or agency, there is a style of intercourse, namely a conversation, that makes the session more palatable to the persons involved. Students particularly have questioned whether the culture makes the difference in the willingness of the client to talk to the worker. Will Native Americans talk as much as whites? Are African-Americans verbal? "After all many of them have not gone to college?" While some of the questions are real inquiries, many are based on stereotypes and prejudicial views of certain groups. Some, of course, come from culture, home, perhaps peers, but unfortunately a great deal come from our profession, its research, and at times its rhetoric.

One revealing example of how professions foment stereotypes about minority groups is presented in an article entitled *Creating a Company of Unequals* (Lorber, 1977). In summary, the agency had set itself up so that clients were categorized and assigned to workers who operated at different levels. The psychiatrists and psychologists were assigned mainly white middle class clients who were verbal and had problems fairly familiar to the middle class, such as problems with a spouse, or a child having a school problem. People with slightly more severe problems, but with some higher education, were assigned to social workers. Multi-problem families, mainly minorities, were assigned to aides and those workers with the least amount of professional training.

Thus, the agency not only loaded down the workers with the least amount of training, giving them problem-saturated clients, but it also set up a status system around which clients were thought to be most desirable, and worthy of the "high-type" helper. In such a situation, could workers not help but feel they were part of a status system? Could they help but think of minorities as less worthy of help?

We would hope that such a situation would not occur in any agency, but could not occur in one oriented to narrative practice. The political nature of the situation would be disclosed, deconstructed, and altered so as to rectify and equalize the assignments. Yes, there might be some cases that would require the skills of the psychiatrist, just as there might be some families who would only need the help the aides provide. But the situations would be dealt with individually, not as a lottery that categorized persons en masse.

While the profession has attempted to deal with aspects of diversity at a level beyond those of most professions, it still is subject to violations of some of its own principles. Efforts to include minorities on boards, committees, and professional offices are important and have been undertaken. At times they have not been just. For example, desirous of having minority leadership in its highest professional offices, some organizations have run a minority against a minority person in order to insure that a minority will win that high office. While they have accomplished their goals they have been manipulative, and insulted the profession by suggesting that it would not elect the capable minority person. While we might applaud the goal, the means by which these well-meaning steps are taken cannot be condoned.

We cannot be expected to differ too strongly from the cultures that envelop us. As Michael White pointed out, we are just as subject to prejudice as others are. Therapeutic situations are not privileged to operate outside of the culture at large. They are not exempt from the structures and from the ideology of the dominant culture. He holds that the therapeutic context is not exempt, it cannot be exempt from the influences and politics of gender, class, race, and culture (White, 1995).

Reflection: As you think about the material you read in this chapter, try to reflect on some of your own ideas and how they may have come to be so important in your life. Are there any beliefs you hold that would be questioned by a person from another cultural group? Are there some cultural values of others that you question? What might be the roots of the different views?

11

Learning and Teaching Narrative Practice

Behold, I do not give lectures or a little charity,
When I give I give myself.

I hear America Singing, the varied carols I hear.

(Walt Whitman)

There is an adventure in learning to practice Narrative Therapy. It is like a trip to a new country, yet with a pentimento of the old country showing through. It is not entirely a strange country. There is a new language to learn, but it is not written with different characters, like Russian or Chinese. You already know some of the customs of the country, regardless of the differences. You know that there is a code of ethics that must be adhered to; you know that the people you work with should be treated with respect and dignity; and you know that it is important to individualize and not to stereotype. If you have had a social work education within the past fifteen years, you have been exposed to a great number of readings on diversity, racism, multiculturalism, discrimination, and the profession's commitment to work for social justice. You have some understanding that context, culture, and environment play an important role in people's lives. You have all been exposed to the idea of the person in the environment, and to the dual perspective.

For most of us the entrance into the arena of a new experience is loaded with opposing emotions. There is the excitement and eagerness to learn something new, which carried us to the experience, but at the same time the fears of risk, criticism, and failure. It is the teacher's job to make the learning situation as positive as possible. Recognizing the dual nature of new experiences, to use that understanding in planning the learning experiences in a way that combines sensitively, with the students' lived experiences.

One of the authors has taught a course on narrative practice for over five years (Narrative Therapy for Social Workers). In addition, there have been numerous workshops and lectures on narrative. What we have found out is that although those involved in the sessions get caught up quickly in the material, it is so simple an idea, yet so alien, compared to what they have been learning in practice, that they wonder if they can ever use it. In addition, it is difficult for them to relate to some of the ideas, particularly externalization.

When we discuss externalization of the problem, for example, there are important questions related to whether or not this lets the client "off the hook" and leads them to believe that their behavior is acceptable. A discussion of what that metaphor means, why we want anyone on the "hook," leads to interesting reflections. Does narrative practice ever suggest that the client is not responsible to work for change? There is always the demand for work, and that is true in a classroom or in the helping situation.

Students who are interns in agencies are concerned that their supervisors are not familiar with the ideas of narrative, and might not accept their attempts to try out any of the ideas. They need to be reassured that they will not have an assignment that would put them in a vulnerable position. It is important to let students know that they are not going to have to use any of these ideas in their field agencies, and that if they do want to try some out it is important to check with their field instructors first. I initiated this procedure after the first year of teaching narrative. We have mentioned the student, who must be an advanced practitioner by now, who decided to send a letter to one of his clients. I was not aware of his actions until I was visited by the field coordinator at the department and asked what "this letter writing was all about." The situation was resolved by examining the narrative concepts with field agencies.

It would be important for the teacher or workshop leader to explain some of the expectations and resistances that they are likely to face. The most important, of course, are the privileged positions some of the current practices hold and the resistance to change. I help the students see the difference early on by asking a simple question, "How many of you have ever thanked your clients?" They are perplexed by this question, but immediately understand that here is a very simple way to recognize the contribution that the client might make to the student's welfare. That is tied together in a mutual effort to help each other give the best service possible. And they also begin to examine how the client might feel knowing that the worker was given to by the client, or offered an idea that might be useful in helping other clients.

Some of the students have thanked clients, and this is discussed with others in the class. Those students who have thanked clients are asked to discuss how they felt when they had been able to announce to the class that they had thanked clients. This led to a discussion of narrative theory and the practice of trying to have an audience for the story telling and the meaning that has for the client. These stories do not necessitate the students talking about themselves at the first meeting, which some students do easily and others with great torment. The class session gets grounded by talking about their meaningful life experiences, not just theory. Furthermore, it helps illustrate the mutual aid involved in the worker/client relationship, and how each needs the other to accomplish their goals. The process is further helped by my pointing out that I cannot be a teacher without a class, and they cannot be a social worker without a client. Each needs the complimentary role in order to fulfill their function. We are tools for each other.

SETTING THE CONTEXT FOR LEARNING: THE SOCIAL WORK CURRICULUM

In the graduate social work program, I usually start off the class with some brief introductions and a little of the philosophy underlying postmodern and deconstructive ideas and how narrative practice relates to them and to social work education and the curriculum. I believe this is important as they tend to see the practice aspect of their training as crucial but other courses as just a necessary evil. Social work programs contain five essential elements which are to be integrated in a manner which demonstrates the total knowledge required for the professional degree. These parts are Human Development and the Social Environment, Policy, Research, and Practice, which includes Field Education. I then present the chart at the top of page 175 for a brief discussion.

In the course of the discussion we look at how narrative practice seems to be an integrating approach which incorporates all of the essentials that might provide a unified approach to practice at all levels. I also point out that other practice approaches could easily make the same claims.

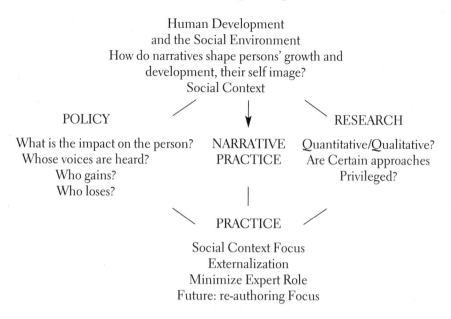

Narrative Practice as a Unifying Concept in Social Work

Human Development
and the Social Environment
How do narratives shape persons' growth and
development, their self image?
Social Context

POLICY   NARRATIVE   RESEARCH

What is the impact on the person?   NARRATIVE   Quantitative/Qualitative?
Whose voices are heard?   PRACTICE   Are Certain approaches
Who gains?   Privileged?
Who loses?

PRACTICE

Social Context Focus
Externalization
Minimize Expert Role
Future: re-authoring Focus

NARRATIVE EXERCISE

One of the major concerns in teaching narrative practice is how to help the person understand the concept of externalization. Unless the person is absolutely new to the helping scene, they may have incorporated an orientation which suggests that they search for the problem, and that often that problem is internal. It is important to help them start to be able to think of the person as separate from the problem. A fairly simple assignment which they can do in about 15 minutes, or take home if it is a class, is the "dragon." This tends to universalize the idea of procrastinating as caused by a dragon, and it is a problem that is not difficult to recognize as something we might all have from time to time. See Figure 11.1.

Although the students are asked to look at their own dragons, many of them will use "procrastination" as their dragon. While at first this was rather frustrating, it soon led to using their responses as a common problem, which many in the class have to combat. It was also seen as an opportunity to use an exercise that Michael White (1995a) has used, where a reporter interviews the "problem," in this case it would be "procrastination" (the dragon) in the presence of a "client" (role-playing) student

"SOMETHING"

On occasion people have been known to ponder on what might keep them from doing certain things, for example, completing a report that was due, or finishing a grant. Persons have been known to say that "something" got in the way, sometimes they know what that something is, a wedding, an illness, lack of time, a broken computer, a test, etc. At other times, they may not know, and might say, most likely to themselves, what's going on, what got in the way? What is that "something"? After years of trying to track down that "something", I believe I have discovered what it is. It is something we believed was extinct, but is in fact still among us. It is a dragon! Now don't laugh, not yet anyway.

Let us imagine that this dragon, named "Something", has certain qualities, qualities which we generally give to humans. It has the ability to think, plan, and it can influence our behavior, perhaps through some magic. Yes, a magic thing which feeds on procrastination. It might help us to think of that thing as a dragon, whose sole effort is to keep us from our work. Of course it is possible that we created this dragon, or at least helped it grow to the point where it can fairly easy keep us in tow. It is sly and magical, like Puff, it can appear to us to be friendly, and let us ride on its back. Or it may be angry, and even though we may not like what it is doing, we might feel it is too powerful for us, all that breathing of fire and smoke. It might even masquerade as a wise dragon at times, convincing us with its wisdom that delay may bring additional knowledge. Never the less, its ultimate goal is to deceive us and have us spend time as its companion.

Dragons have been around a long time and have figured out many ways to conjure us into procrastination. Now one thing else about that "thing" whatever it is out there. It tends to increase in power each time we delay, it savors the victory and weakens our belief that we have the power to deal with that thing. We begin to feel that it is easier to let the "thing" have its way then to battle it.

But all is not lost, history shows that people have found ways to conquer dragons and to deal with those "things" which try to make us believe they have power over us. One strategy is to join with others and attack the thing by finding out how people have dealt with it in the past. Another dragon slayer keeps a record of what seems to help overcome that "something", under what conditions does s/he beat it, and when does it win. What circumstances permit it to take over. For example, when you know a paper is due, and that "thing" starts to urge you to let it go awhile, or go to the library next week, rather then today, or not outline the paper, or set aside time. What do you say and do to the thing which helps it win, what do you do or say to it that overcomes its malevelant advice.

There are many things that happen which get in our way and we can decide whether or not it is dragon smoke blown in our faces, or serious incidents that warrant setting aside other tasks. There are consequences that need to be considered. But there are some "things" which are not "really" real, and become excuses which that "something" has planted to undermine our efforts. That "thing" needs to be cornered. We can seek strategies to combat "Something", the dragon; we can find out what works, and once more save humanity from those fire breathing monsters.

FIGURE 11.1 Dragon exercise.

who has said procrastination is his/her dragon. A student volunteers to be the person suffering from the problem, another the dragon, "procrastination," who the reporter interviews, asking questions such as:

How did you come to be an expert of procrastination?
Are there some persons you find easier to recruit into procrastination than others are?
Who are the most difficult?
What are the situations that permit you to function best?
Off the record now, what works in resisting your recruitment?
What makes you so hard to resist?
Are there any protections against procrastination?

The reporter, or the class, can interview the person who is listening to the problem and ask him/her to speak and ask questions about what s/he learned, or might do now. He/she could also ask, "What experiences did the other group members notice about their own lives during this exercise? What about the person's story affected those experiences?"

Freedman and Combs (1996) have an excellent externalizing exercise. It contains two parts. In the first, the reader is given the following instructions:

"Note the overall effect of answering these questions. How do you feel? What seems possible in regard to the "Pick a character trait, quality, or emotion that you feel you have too much of or that other people sometimes complain about in you." Make sure it is in adjective form, as a description of you, for instance "angry, competitive," "guilty," or "nitpicky." In the following set of questions, fill in the trait of emotion where we have an "X." As you read these questions, substituting the trait or emotion for X, answer them to yourself.

1. How did you become X?
2. What are you most "X" about?

What kinds of things happen that typically lead to your being X? Is it a trait or emotion?
What seems impossible? How does the future look in regard to this?"

A number of other questions follow and then the participants are asked to proceed to the second portion of the assignment.

In the second part, they are asked to,

"Take the same quality or trait that you worked with above and make it into a noun. For example if "X" was "competitive," it would now become "competition"; "angry" would become "anger." In the following questions, where we've written a "Y," fill in your noun. . . ." They are also asked to reflect on the same questions as above.

1. What made you vulnerable to the Y so that it was able to dominate your life?
2. In what contexts is the Y likely to take over?"

As in the first part there are additional questions.

There is then a discussion related to the differences in feelings and sense of the future as well as which made you feel like an object (pp. 49–50).

When I use this exercise I insist that no names be put on the document, and students discuss their feeling in general as they wish following the exercise, looking particularly at comparing the two parts. The following is one person's responses to that exercise.

The XY Exercise

X. Guilty

1. I became guilty very young because of not being able to fulfill the expectations I thought I should.
2. I am most guilty about family, husband, children, parents, in-laws and outlaws, sometimes clients.
3. I am guilty when I feel I've failed somebody. . . .
4. When I am guilty I try to make amends. I worry, I don't sleep well. I forget myself.
5. Just about everything I have done has a relationship to feeling guilty.
6. . . .
7. When I'm guilty I feel inadequate and inept.
8. If I were not guilty, I could look out for what I want and stop forgetting who I am.

Comments: I feel ashamed of how much of my life has been dominated by guilty feelings. It seems as if I'm stuck with it because it is so much part of me and the best I can do is manage it more successfully.

Y: Guilt

1. I became vulnerable to guilt because during the war I couldn't help my mother feel better when she was sad and lonely.
2. Whenever someone I am close to has a problem.

It continues with other responses and reporting on and comparing X and Y impact.

The use of case material, even when it has not been set up in the narrative style, offers the participants opportunities to reflect on how they would handle the situation from a narrative practice perspective. The case of Laura is such an opportunity. Laura is faced with so many problems it is fair to say she is problem-saturated. The participant is asked "What's the matter with Laura?" They are asked to write her a letter assuming that they have obtained the information in the case material. How is not the question. This assignment is usually given after they have had some exposure to the idea of externalization of the problem. The purpose is to examine how they select from the areas of concern that Laura expressed to externalize the problem. Some excerpts follow.

> Dear Laura, I enjoyed getting to know you at our first meeting. Here is my understanding of what we talked about. I'd like you to let me know next meeting if anything sounds wrong, or if I left out anything that is important . . . You have really been very brave in facing nasty situations . . . (continues).
>
> Dear Laura, First I want to say how glad I am your grandmother brought you to see me today. She cares about you and wants you to go to school.
>
> From your story it is clear that some of the things you have had to cope with have been terribly difficult. Some of the adults in your life have not cared for you and protected you as you deserve. I am impressed by how you have survived the hardship and painful experiences you have had . . . I want you to remember that you have shown a great deal of sense and will power in many of the ways you have coped with your difficulties . . . (continues).

LETTER WRITING

Presenting some vignette material, or their questions about a client they are working with, and asking the students to write a brief letter they might send following the meeting they had. Those that wish, read the letters in class. Some of the class members are asked to be a reflecting team and react to some of the points made, and comment on how their own experiences (letters) compared to the reader's. An example:

Dear Mr. F.

I hope this note finds you feeling more comfortable these days. I am enjoying getting to know you better. When we talked yesterday, you shared
some of your life experiences, including your harrowing adventures in
combat during the war . . . Looking at all the greeting cards your children
have given you I am struck by the support for you here at (an institution).
They must have gotten a great deal from you as a father.

Following the readings, reflecting groups of class members may be
asked to respond and write their own letters as a group.

REFLECTING GROUPS

When a video or film is shown, class members rotate as a reflecting group
to respond to some of the things that they noted in the presentation. The
remainder of the class can then react to the group's comments and to
the video.

ROLE PLAY

Vignettes and short sketches are presented to the class and they are asked
to role-play the situation. The materials vary from a middle class family
with two children, one with behavior problems at school; a mother on
welfare who needs housing; a person with alcohol problems who has lost
three jobs in the past year; a gang group in trouble with the law.

GENOGRAMS

We have used these in many ways as a brief assignment to be handed in
quickly with a one- or two-generation plotting or more complicated
requirements.

The latter assignment, a three-generation contextual genogram, is
time demanding, and is best used in a class with an extended time period
(2–3 months). These are different from the usual genograms because the
students are asked to check with some of the people on the genogram to
try to find out from them what the contextual, historical events were that
most shaped their lives at various times in their life histories. For some of

the students who have had to contact parents, grandparents, and other relatives, it has been, in their words, a revelation.

Here is a situation where the student's story gets to be shaped by the assignment. They find out that some of the things they have been told are not the truth, or at least there are a number of versions of the truth. In fact, that one can rewrite history all the time. For example, finding out that you are adopted rewrites your past history. In addition, they get to see just how important context can be—wars, job opportunities, the depression, and television bursting on the scene are some of the contextual events that seem to have shaped their ancestors' lives.

Students are given the opportunity to discuss their genograms in class to the extent that they wish. Many are interested in sharing and hearing others' stories. The class begins to recognize just how important stories are in the lives of all persons. They also begin to discuss commonalities in the lives that seem to cross race and class lines. For example, many of the students will talk about how their parents are still fearful of spending money, a carryover from their experiences during the depression. A number talk of how a loss during the war impacted the direction their family took, or how the search for jobs led them to leave their home for the states, or for a foreign country.

The assignment starts to bring the class together as they share their experiences, an unanticipated outcome of the assignments which have now been incorporated in the expectations of the students' reporting. The genogram (see Figure 11.2) is a tool that they also feel they can use with clients, regardless of the practice approach they privilege.

NARRATIVE WORKBOOK

In addition to the readings the students are presented with a workbook, *Reflections on Narrative Therapy*, that is to be completed by the end of the semester. Some of the items they are asked to respond to are:

In a number of fields, writers say that Narratives help people make sense of their lives, how does that work?

What are the main ideas that White uses from Foucault's philosophy?

What makes the use of externalization such a powerful helping tool?

Illustrate the concept of "mapping the influence of a problem" in the case of a teenager on drugs.

Why might it be accurate to consider Narrative Therapy a therapy of liberation? In what ways is it not accurate?

Families exist in time, and the genogram helps us understand a particular cohort based on events in the historical time of that person.

Part 1. DUE _____

Prepare a three generation Genogram of you and your family.

*In addition to the general information, give the approximate year of birth and the place if known.

For each generation, what major nationals or world events or developments in the first 25 years of their lives might have shaped their lives, i.e. the Depression, invention of TV, wars, immigration. If you are able, interview one of the people in each generation and ask them what might have influences the direction of their lives. Are there any important stories they would like to tell? What did you learn that you didn't know about your family?

Part 2. DUE _____

Prepare a similar Genogram for another family (client, friend, neighbor, etc.). This should be entirely free, open and unformed request.

Try to obtain information as above.

Part 3.

Discuss and compare your first Genogram with the second.

(If this assignment is in any way a difficult one for personal reasons, please discuss with me and we can arrange a different assignment.)

FIGURE 11.2   Genogram assignment.

There are a total of twenty-two questions, and in part they reflect the time line of the course. This serves as their final paper. It is collected once about one-third through the course. It is not graded at that time, but feedback is given as to whether or not it meets the requirements.

LEARNING AND TEACHING IN SUPERVISION

There is a tradition of supervision in social work. It is related in part to the idea of accountability to the agency and usually a particular person for the quality of one's work. Furthermore, the intensity in the nature of the problems dealt with and the large numbers of cases requires the opportunity to share experiences, seek information, make comparisons among approaches, and get credit for one's work. The worker is not alone. Often, workers with a great deal of experience seek consultation with other workers about some of their cases, while supervision has generally followed the model of a person with more experience helping a person with less experience learn how to do their job in an effective and satisfying manner. We would see this just a little differently; it need not be a person with more experience, but someone who can help a person reflect on what they are doing.

In a previous document we defined supervision as: "The process by which people assist each other in learning the skills, attitudes and knowledge needed to perform their function in the agency in an effective and satisfying manner" (Abels, 1977a).

At that time, I was advocating that the role of the supervisor needed to change from "the" expert or overseer, a person with super-vision, to supervisor as counselor in a "reciprocal transaction within the agency system . . . a synergist who helps unite divergent views and helps locate new knowledge to be 'synthesized with the old into a greater whole.'" This synergistic approach unites people by minimizing "the statuses and differences that separate them" (Abels, 1977a).

This was in contrast to some of the supervisor as expert views at that time. For example, supervision as ". . . an educational process in which a person with certain equipment of knowledge and skill takes responsibility for training a person with less equipment" (Robinson, 1930)

One of the important things to consider when helping a worker look at a new practice approach is how much of the person is invested in the "doing" they have incorporated into their way of helping. They are often secure with the approach they use, and even though they may be eager to learn something new, there will be doubts and resistances. Narrative cannot be pushed, but some of the techniques that the worker is trying to learn should be reflected in the approach to supervision.

If the worker brings up the issue of not having time to really read some of the material, or to write a letter, and so forth, then the discussion might suggest that "overwork" is getting in the way of him/her using the narrative approach. This is not "caseworking" the worker, but a way of challenging the obstacles to the use of the narrative framework by using a narrative approach to do so.

Group supervision of staff, in which the staff becomes a reflecting team when a case is discussed, is also another way narrative can be reflected in supervision. Some of the guidelines on how a narrative team operates differently from the usual concept of team feedback can be discussed.

For students, the group also provides a security of numbers, and the recognition that others are in the same boat. For beginning learners, there is also the respite from being away from responsibility for clients, makes learning easier.

The supervisor's refusal to be the expert, the "answer man or woman" further illustrates the belief in the narrative approach. The supervisee must become their own consultant as far as possible.

Some of the same exercises that were used in the class can be used in supervision. While I would not ask a worker to do a personal genogram, as it may be too uncomfortable to share their history, they might examine a client's genogram and get an understanding of how historical context influences a person's actions and beliefs. It would be important to discuss how they would have felt if I had asked for their genogram and parallel that with concerns the client might have about doing a genogram, or we might discuss our own genogram.

Viola Spolin's book *Improvisation for the Theater* provides a number of excellent exercises which deal with communication listening sensitivity, connections, and self understanding. The authors have used these over the years with students and have found them stimulating, fun, and appreciated by the students. Spolin who had been active in the early development of Chicago's "Second City Company" had been influenced by Neva Boyd's teaching of social group work (Spolin, 1963).

CONCLUSION: ABOUT LEARNING AND TEACHING

Reynolds suggested that there are stages in the learning process that are important for a teacher (supervisor) to understand if they are going to be helpful to the learner (Reynolds, 1934, pp. 75–85). These five stages will just be outlined briefly:

1. *The stage of acute consciousness of self.* This is similar to stage fright, and to not knowing what to do. The role of the teacher here is to offer security.
2. *The stage of sink-or-swim adaptation.* There is some inkling of what needs to be done—the role of the teacher is to help the person integrate the learning and mobilize the skills the person already has.

3. *The stage of understanding the situation without power to control one's own activity in it.* Less of a concern with self. Illumination about what to do, difficulty in doing it. The teacher helps the person be honest about what they did, why it worked or did not work.

4. *The stage of relative mastery, in which one can both understand and control one's activity in the art which is to be learned.* Not as much need for a teacher, other than to acknowledge their "professionalization," help the person think about research, and understand that there is always more to be learned as a professional.

5. *The stage of learning to teach what one has mastered.* Helping the person understand that teaching will set in motion for them the same stage process that they went through in learning narrative. New challenges present some of the same growth challenges.

I would like to close this chapter with a quotation from the work of Bertha Reynolds (1934).

. . . you can always trust a group to teach you what you may teach them." The statement is met with incredulity at first. The skills necessary to evoke from a group this revelation of their needs are not inconsiderable. (Compare the skills needed to help a client in casework to make clear his/her needs.) At first these skills seem unattainable. Soon, however— very soon if the leader is capable of some trust in people even when the outcome is in doubt—a group begins to respond and to make itself known. The joy of seeing that a relationship of trust actually works is second to no other joy in a teacher's life. (p. 120)

12

Liberating Practice

Alice (In Wonderland) asks:
"Would you tell me, please, which way I ought to go from here?"
"That depends a good deal on where you want to get to," said the cat.
"I don't much care," said Alice.
"Then it doesn't matter which way you go," said the cat.
"So long as I get *somewhere*," Alice added as an explanation.
"Oh, your sure to do that," said the Cat, "if you only walk long enough."

Lewis Carol

"And I know, too, that we must keep endless watch on ourselves lest in a careless moment we breath in somebody's face and fasten the infection on him. What's natural is the microbes. All the rest-health, integrity, purity (if you like)—is a product of human will, of a vigilance that must never falter. The good man, the man who infects hardly anyone, is the man who has the fewest lapses of attention. And it needs tremendous willpower, a never ending tension of the mind to avoid such lapses." (p. 229)

(The Plague, Albert Camus)

THE REFLECTIVE PRACTITIONER

In Albert Camus' *The Plague* (1991), Tarrou and Dr. Rieux take an hour off from their voluntary struggle against the pestilence to reflect about the world around them, and Tarrou tells the story of his life. He has discovered through his various experiences that no one on earth is free from the plague. The Plague can be seen as a metaphor for prejudice and discrimination (Kellman, 1985, pp. 47–49).

The reflective practitioner thinks not only about the process and the results, but also about the consequences of actions of those one works with, as well as for him/herself. The demand on professionals to know themselves, as well as to use themselves in the helping process, is a vital one. This type of reflection can lead to enlightened and enhanced practice. At the heart of narrative practice is a strong commitment to treat the client with the utmost respect, to minimize diagnostic assessments, and to relate to the lived experience of the client. The cultural mandates of a particular group are important to consider because they can both support and retard the helping process (Holland & Kilpatrick, 1993). It is important to note that some of the cultural mandates may indeed be the problem (Mumby, 1994; Langellier, 1994), such as the treatment of women in some traditional conservative religious groups. Susann Moller Okin speaks to this subject cogently in an article entitled, *Is Multiculturalism Bad for Women?* (Okin, 1999). Some cultures, she maintains, have as one of their principle aims the control of women by men. At the worst of times, women are not only marginalized, but used as pawns in war. This can lead to being ostracized from their communities and at times suicide.

The worker as expert needs to assess him/herself, and will be assessed; it is clear that the worker as an "outsider" can rarely understand another person's culture and its impact on that person (Reynolds, 1934). This is particularly true when the worldview of the helper is vastly different from that of the person seeking help. But the workers can constantly ask themselves whether they are imposing their own story onto the client. In a sense, workers must liberate themselves from their own cultural biases and their own traditional therapy stories.

Francis Fanon (1967) spoke about this, in relation to his experiences in Algeria in the early 1950s when Algeria was still a French colony. As a psychiatrist trained in the west, he attempted to make his helping relevant to the Algerian people (Gordon, 1996). Our profession has taken leadership, historically and on the present scene, in acknowledging the importance of cross-cultural sensitivity, but we have not yet evolved the practice that compliments our understanding. We have at times punished those in our profession who have professed a more radical action oriented practice. This was true for Bertha Capen Reynolds in the 1940s, and Harry Specht in the 1990s. His position in his book *Fallen Angels* (1993) was attacked on many occasions by some clinically oriented workers, who saw a call for more social action as an attack on their practice. I recall one social work conference in California at which I introduced him and he spoke about his book. The major audience reaction was the defense of clinical practice. In many ways we have become captive to a particular mode of practice supported by powerful forces in the profession who have used methods such as licensing and accreditation to privilege certain practice approaches and subjugate knowledge of others. These processes serve as important professional safeguards for clients, but have also been used for personal privilege and advantage. Feeling that their voices have not been heard, groups within the profession, such as group work and community organization, have formed their own organizations.

We see the narrative perspective as one that is liberating (Abels & Abels, 1997). It strives to liberate the person from being the problem, or being saturated by the problem. It furthermore is liberating in that it expands the participant's ability to recognize the limitations that have been placed on him/her by social forces. It liberates them by helping them find ways to rewrite their stories. It is liberating in that it offers a broader view of their historical subplots. It is liberating to the worker because it supports the idea that s/he does not have to have the answers to all problems, and is not an expert. It is liberating because it deals with the person's entire lived experience in the landscape of their lives. It recognizes the importance of providing the client with new knowledge, and that in itself is liberating.

It liberates the profession from the bonds of having a practice either for work with individuals and a different practice for working with groups and communities. It liberates by unifying the profession with an approach that is useful overall. It liberates by reminding us that we need not be the expert knowing all the answers, and liberates us to search and inquire after new knowledge. It liberates us from making decisions on behalf of the client that hopefully can have good outcomes, but diminish the person's own agency.

I would like to examine the situation where Salvador Minuchin, working with a mother in family therapy, signed off for her. This kept her from having her child taken from her by the welfare department, but it also meant that he took responsibility for her behavior. This presents some interesting insights into the current situation in the mental health area. Since he "signed off" on her, he has power over her. She will have to meet certain conditions, which he may not have set, but which he will attempt to enforce. In a sense they both have power over each other. Of course it is not equal power, and she could suffer the loss of her child, yet what he did was a moral act (Minuchin, 1991).

It is that type of power and control that Foucault was concerned about and wrote about. Since no psychiatrist is going to be in a position to watch the client at all times, in fact only for a small portion of time, techniques have to be developed that provide for self monitoring by the client. He refers to this as: "Internalized personal discourse . . . an action of self-control guided by set social standards" (Foucault, 1982). He suggests, "people monitor and conduct themselves according to their interpretations of set cultural norms and may also seek out central authority figures such as a religious leader or psychoanalyst for further guidance" (Madigan, 1996, p. 268).

As part of his premise about control Foucault (1977) referred to Jeremy Bentham's Panoptican (1791). This was a proposed prison where the inmates were arranged in ways so that they could be observed by the guards who they could not see, but never knew if the guard was watching them, so they would be prone to behave at all times (see Figure 12.1). He proposed it as a means of social reform. He believed that this would encourage exemplary behavior at all times (Barton, 1993). Wrongdoing did not often require more punishment than the "gaze" which is a cultural way of indicating displeasure. It works, as most children, students, and subordinates know.

Another form society provides for self-monitoring is the use of drugs. This has become a valuable, though often over-used method of helping people lead fairly normal lives. Making the client return weekly to a Methadone maintenance clinic or to an office to receive their "meds" is a form of social control. It serves both as a control function and monitoring function to help the person regulate their own behavior and get in the habit of taking their "meds." The major difficulty is that often persons on those mediating drugs begin to believe they are better, perhaps cured, and go off their "meds." They than regress and end up in an institution of some kind. Another concern is that the drugs often become a substitute for the more expensive conversations with a helper that may alleviate the problem. The person's story continues to be drug-related. While this may be necessary in some cases, it may not be the treatment of choice for all.

Drugs have been used in negative ways as a source of control. One example was the heavy importation of opium into China by foreign countries in order to keep the population from resisting foreign takeovers. This led to the opium wars.

THE MORALITY PLAY'S THE THING

A recent film, *The Truman Show*, is the story of a young man who discovers his entire life has been staged with him as the central figure in a three-decade long television show. *Truman* is a True-Man in that he is unaware of the way he is being used. He is not a True-Man because all of

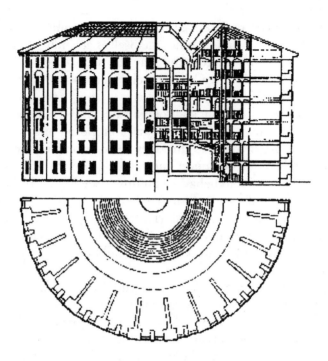

FIGURE 12.1   The Panopticon of Jeremy Bentham. From Barton and Barton, *Modes of Power in Technical and Professional Visuals*, p. 139.

the experiences he faces are "set-ups," seemingly real, but artificial experiences, with primed people/actors, who follow a script and not their own direction. He alone is doing what is natural, of course, natural within the limits being set by a conspiracy of actions. All of his problems are resolved and worked out for him by others. But, of course, his problems are also created by others; they are scripted. Persons grow through the ability to work on the problems they face, and so he must face problems, and of course this gives tension to his life which is much appreciated by the millions who watch the program. Truman is not permitted to search out his own solutions to problems. When things get too rough, a new character is introduced into the scenario, a long lost teenage sweetheart, an actress who abandoned her written lines and tried to warn *Truman* that he was really on TV. Unknown to him, his desires and plans are all deliberately thwarted, and he is forced to live the life others provide for him.

A series of technical errors alerts him to the fact that he is not in control of his life. Ultimately, and against great odds, he breaks out of the lifelong narrative that has been selected for him, out to the world, "less safe" perhaps, but a world in which he will have the right to his own self-fulfillment, and be able to make his own moral decisions. As the movie closes we see his once teenage love running to meet him. As he walks out of the dome in which his life was shaped, the scene shifts to TV audiences all over the world cheering. It is a like a universal morality play, and True-Man, "*Everyman*," has chosen freedom. The confused, but enthralled world which has enjoyed his enslavement, and their own, by the way, for almost thirty years, glories in his freedom, not realizing their own conspiratorial guilt or personal enslavement. One might hope that his experience was a lesson learned, but in the closing scene with *The Truman Show* off the air the viewers just switch a channel to another program. The movie is a good illustration of Foucault's concern with both power and subjugated knowledge. Truman was a victim of both.

Like the television audience in *The Truman Show*, the helping professions may, though unaware of it, be performers in processes controlled by some prime movers in our society whose orientation toward human needs is self-centered and manipulative, and who often lack the "empathy" that Goleman speaks to in his work *Emotional Intelligence* (Goleman, 1998). This unawareness on our part is often at a cost to the clients and perhaps to ourselves as well.

For the healing professions, those concerned with social justice, empathy is a given and we know that all decisions that we make concerning our clients, are moral decisions, that is, we are always trying to decide on what is the right thing to do. We are always actors in a morality play. The things we do or do not do make a difference in people's lives. The narratives in this book reflect that idea. Our morality play's actors, the physicians, the social workers, the mental health professionals, and the teachers, reveal their inner thoughts about their moral dilemmas, many of which are created by the restrictions placed on them by powerful interests that can set the conditions for their practice. Dissatisfaction with some HMO's which curtailed physicians' ability to serve have created a growing protest from patients, and a movement by doctors to turn to unions, in an attempt to counteract the controls being placed on their ability to give needed service. Limiting service is seen by these doctors as a moral issue, particularly when the laws on the issues are illusive or enhanced by contracts they are committed to sign. All of us, physicians and patients alike, are captive to the morality of the organization. We have seen traditional public services made private and some organizations' policies change from caring to "privateering."

Madigan (1993) points out that as a therapist, "White acts to liberate persons from dominant knowledge and power practices. He acts with purpose in proposing that persons become linguistically radicalized against them. For example, he would juxtapose the scientific or media-driven story of the person with the person's unique account story of themselves" (p. 277).

Current self-monitoring methods are increasing in the work place where staff using the Internet are monitored, at times not aware of the monitoring. Some have been told that all of their communications will be recorded in some way. This served to limit their use of the web, and they monitor themselves. The ability to listen in on what radio and TV programs a person is attending to has also served as a self-monitoring device. Some of it is used for commercial purposes, to sell products, and at times to correct certain errors a person has made in ordering goods, and so on.

Back in 1973, before the postmodern movement began, and prior to any ideas about Narrative Therapy, Allen Wheelis (1973), a psychiatrist, wrote:

> Since freedom depends on awareness, psychotherapy may by extending awareness, create freedom. But not surely, and not always. When in therapy a life story is examined in such a way that the patient knows and feels, what he remembers and can reason from, is systematically discounted, while significant causality is located only in those unconscious forces postulated by the therapist, in hidden constraints situational and libidinal which allegedly twisted him and shaped defenses, required that he react in the way he did and in no other—all in this one is rewriting the past, is taking a story which must have contained elements of freedom and responsibility and retelling it in terms of only causes lying outside awareness and hence beyond control; so teaching the patient to see himself as the passive product of inscrutable knowledge. Where he feels himself to be the author of action, his analysis will show him to be "acting out," that is, an object being acted upon. (p. 113)

In this paragraph we find the concepts that could be a foundation for Narrative Therapy, the idea of the life story; the discounting of the client's views; worker as expert; the client as an object; the subjugation of knowledge; and the rewriting. All on behalf of searching for freedom. Although trained in the modernist perspective as an analyst, he speaks like a postmodernist:

> In reconstructing a life story truth is necessary but not sufficient. Truth does not demarcate, and cannot determine whether we would dwell upon

cause of choice. Two histories of the same life may be radically different, yet equally true. If we have failed an examination we may say, "I would not have failed if the teacher had not asked that question on Cromwell, which, after all, had not come up in class," or "I would not have failed if I had studied harder." Both the statements are addressed to the same experience, in the same effort to understand; both claim to answer the question "Why did I fail?" and both may be true. Truth does not here provide the criterion for selection; the way we understand the past is determined, rather by the future we desire." (Wheelis, p. 115)

Both his considerations of what is the truth, and his comments on how we select the parts of the story to fit our desired futures might be right out of a narrative philosophical framework. One final reference to Wheelis's work,". . . in the life most crushed by outside forces there is nevertheless the potentiality for actions other than those taken. With the noose around our necks there are still options—to curse God or to pray, to weep or to slap the executioner in the face (pp. 115–116).

Wheelis had all of the theoretical stance that is congruent with the social constructive philosophies that support narrative practice, yet he did not put those ideas together into a practice framework. It may be that the contextual forces in society at that time were not yet ready. Or was it the same phenomena that kept Avebury (Michell, 1983) hidden from view. All the pieces were visible but the gestalt was not visible until a particular lens made sense of the pieces.

In discussing the awareness that we gain through the helping process, Wheelis condemns the idea that the unconscious forces be postulated as determining causes which remain outside our experience. He says "If, however, the determining causes of which we gain awareness, lie within, or are brought within, our experience, and if we use this gain in understanding to create present options, freedom will be increased, and with it greater responsibility for what we have been, are, and will become" (p. 117).

There is still a great deal of work to be done before narrative practice gains the support that it needs to impact some of the more traditional bastions of practice theory. Its minimizing need for assessments and labels complicates things for practitioners who would like to use the approach, but who need to make a diagnosis in keeping with the DSM standards.

It is a problem as well for those who firmly believe that the person needs to see himself or herself as the problem. They will find it most difficult to accept the concept of externalization. Some claim it gets the client "off the hook," as if clients were a fish that we hooked. Those who hold that a worker needs to give instructions, assignments, and develop a strategy for the client will not want to create the situation where the client sets their own directions. Those who feel that to a large degree the motivation to change is related to seeing the worker as an expert will find it irreverent for a worker to take a "know nothing" stance.

Some of the criticism of Narrative Therapy deserves careful concern. It is not a perfect entity, but a complex evolving and dynamic approach open to new ideas and modification. Salvadore Minuchin, for example, after attending some workshops in which he observed narrative therapists at work, was concerned that narrative, ". . . does not require working with the family. This made me wonder whether the postmodernist ideas that seem so prevalent in the literature of the field had anything to do with the disappearance of the family from the therapeutic process" (Minuchin, 1998, p. 397).

He believes that the attention paid to the political nature of social constructionist theory did not deal with the relationship among family members. "In other words can a narrative therapist work with the family as a social system" (p. 399)? He may also be evaluating the broader concern expressed by some narrative therapists, that systems thinking is too structured, narrow, and restrictive a concept, a belief held by some social workers as well (Wakefield, 1996). Minuchin believes that the importance of family as context requires work with the family members as a unit in order to involve the relationship aspects of the family, and these may be missing in narrative practice.

In the same journal issue, are the responses to Minuchin by Gene Combs and Jill Freedman in *Tellings and Retellings*, Karl Tomm in *A Question of Perspective*, Carlos E. Sluzki in *In Search of the Lost Family: A Footnote to Minuchin's Essay*. These make for an interesting extension of the ideas of narrative practice (*Journal of Marriage and Family Therapy*, 1998, 24(4).

What the questioning by Minuchin has served to do is to bring Narrative Therapy more into the awareness of those in the helping profession who had not been aware or interested in it. As one of the historic contributors to family work his involvement with narrative serves to keep the dialogue alive. It is important as well, because as a scientist/therapist he is working in the tradition of inquiry and the pursuit of the "best" approach to helping.

"Where will all of the deconstructive efforts go?" Lynn Hoffman suggests that at least for her, it is time for "Setting Aside the Model in Family Therapy." She writes, "Does this mean that I am throwing out larger theories of knowledge along with models? No, I am only reconstructing them for their own good. As long as they are 'paradigms,' which means useful pots to put things in, they are necessary (Hoffman, 1998)."

Not sure yet what the future may bring, her writing would suggest that the reflective practitioner could make use of many forms of help from metaphor, art, writing, poetry. She lauds Michael White, stating that,

> What White has done in general is to naturalize therapy. If the therapeutic boundary were shaky before, it has now collapsed. White goes directly into the lives of those consulting with him, ignoring the caste lines of traditional mental health . . . White tries to create for people what he calls a community of concern and I call an attending community . . . Finally, I want to mention a less tangible element of White's style, which I call 'withness.' He is careful not to engage in any move without checking it out. 'Is this alright with you?' is a frequent question. (pp. 151–152)

It was these innovations in practice style that led to Hoffman's considering that it may be time to set aside the models. What she saw in Michael White's work, and in Narrative Therapy, is what we saw. It was a "natural" way to help people. We are reminded that our one time childhood hero was not Paul Bunyon who seemed against nature, but John Henry who was "with the people, and about whom people sang."

> John Henry said to his captain
> A man is Just a man
> He was a steel driving man
> He was a natural man

A FINAL WORD

We have presented some of the ideas of narrative that we believe embodied the soul of its contribution. We have done so in a manner aimed at stimulating your interest in an approach to helping which we believe both liberates us as helpers and those with whom we work. We have tried to emphasize the efforts of social workers and their contributions to narrative practice. Our presentation, however, cannot substitute for the understanding you will get by going to the readings and videotapes of Michael White and David Epston.

The continuing struggle of freedom versus control is one with which social workers are familiar. The values of the profession have been those which hold with the rights of clients to live their lives, to receive help, and to use it as they will with the least possible control or interference in their life narrative. This has been a continuous battle waged against those who hold the giving of funds or services allows the imposition of controls over the lives of clients and the imposition of the giver's narrative. We must constantly renew our belief in freedom and equality. Listening carefully to the client's story permits us, as it did Walt Whitman, to hear America singing its varied carols, and to recognize that the heart of narrative therapy is not stasis, but transformation. There are new carols to be heard.

References

Abels, P. (1969). Riding with batman, superman, and the green hornet: Experiences in a very special group. *Mental Retardation, 7*(1), 37–39.

Abels, P. (1971). Instructed advocacy and community groupwork. *Social work practice: Conference on Social Welfare.* New York: Columbia University Press.

Abels, P. (1973). The managers are coming! The managers are coming! *Public Welfare, 31*(4), 13–15.

Abels, P. (1977a). *The new practice of supervision and staff development: A synergistic approach.* New York: Association Press.

Abels, P. (1977b). Terra incognita: The future of the profession, *Social Work, 20*(1), 25–28.

Abels, P. (1984). *Mediating the stress of serious illness in the inner-city.* Presentation, National Conference on Social Work. Washington, D.C.

Abels, P. (1997a). Can ethnic agencies more effectively serve ethnic communities than mainstream agencies? In D. de Anda (Ed.), *Controversial issues in Multiculturalism.* Boston: Allyn and Bacon.

Abels, P. (1997b). Voices from the depths. *Reflections: Narratives of Professional Helping, 3*(3), 2–3.

Abels, P., & Abels, S. L. (1997, October). *Narrative therapy in group work: The practice of liberation.* Paper presented at the Association for the Advancement of Social Work with Groups. Quebec, Canada.

Abels, P., & Abels, S. L. (1999, October). *Narrative practice: Just in time.* Paper presented at the Association for the Advancement of Social Work with Groups Conference. Denver, CO.

Abels, P., & Murphy, M. (1981). *Administration in the human services.* Englewood Cliffs, NJ: Prentice Hall.

Abels, P., & Oliver, J. (1997, April). *Voices not heard.* Paper presented at Poverty Conference. California State University, Long Beach, CA.

Abels, S. L. (1995). Editorial. *Reflections: Narratives of Professional Helping, 1*(1), 2–3.

Abels, S. L., & Abels, P. (1980). Social group work's contextual purposes. *Social Work With Groups, 3*(2), 1–12.

Abels, S. L., & Abels, P. (1986). Social group work. In A. Fink, J. Pfouts, & A. Dobelstein (Eds.), *The field of social work* (pp. 198–221). Beverly Hills: Sage.

Abels, S. L., & Abels, P. (2000, October). *Social connectiveness: Social work's mission.* Paper presented at the Association for the Advancement of Social Work with Groups, Toronto, Canada.

Adams-Wescott, J., & Denbart, I. (1995). A journey of change through connection. In S. Friedman, *The reflecting team in action.* New York: Guilford.

Addams, J. (1935). *Twenty years at Hull House.* New York: McMillan.

Anderson, H. (1997). *Conversation, language, and possibilities: A postmodern approach to therapy.* New York: Basic Books.

Anderson, H. (1999). Reimagining family therapy: Reflections on Minuchin's invisible family. *Journal of Marital and Family Therapy, 25*(1), 1–8.

Anderson, T. (1991). *The reflecting team.* New York: Norton.

Bacigalupe, G. (1996). Writing in therapy: A participatory approach. *Journal of Family Therapy, 18*(4), 361–373.

Bandura, A. (1989). Human agency in social cognitive theory. *American Psychologist, 44*(9), 1175–1184.

Barton, B. F., & Barton, S. M. (1993). Modes of power in technical and professional visuals. *JBTC, 7*(1), 138–162.

Barry, D. (1997). Telling changes: From narrative family therapy to organizational change & development. *Journal of Organizational Change Management, 10*(1), 32–48.

Bateson, G. (1972). *Steps to an ecology of the mind.* New York: Ballantine.

Beito, D. T. (2000). *From mutual aid to the welfare state.* Chapel Hill, NC: University of North Carolina Press.

Bentham, J. (1791). *Panopticon: Postscript part II.* London: T. Payne.

Besa, D. (1994). Narrative family therapy: A multiple baseline outcome study including collateral effects on verbal behavior. *Research in Social Work Practice, 43*(3), 309–325.

Borden, W. (1992). Narrative perspectives in psychosocial interventions following adverse life events. *Social Work, 37*(2), 135–139.

Bracho, A. (2000). An institute of community participation. *Dulwich Centre Journal, 6,* 6–16.

Bridgitte, Sue, Mem, & Veronica. (1996, Summer). Power to our journeys. *AFTA Newsletter,* 1–16. Dulwich Center, Adelaide, So. Australia.

Brower, A. M. (1996). Group development as constructed social reality revisited: The constructivism of small groups. *Families in Society: The Journal of Contemporary Human Services, 77*(6), 336–344.

Brozann, N. (1999, March 2). *New York Times,* p. D7.

Bruner, J. (1990). *Acts of meaning.* Cambridge, MA: Harvard University Press.

Bruner, J. S. (1991). The narrative construction of reality. *Critical Inquiry, 18,* 1–21.

Bulhan, H. A. (1985). *Franz Fanon and the psychology of oppression.* New York: Plenum Press.

Buss, T. (1989). Misrepresenting health and human service agency caseload data: Problems and solutions. *Journal of Human Health Resource Administration,* 342–351.

Camus, A. (1991). *The plague.* New York: Vintage International.

Caplan, G. (1974). *Support systems and community mental health.* New York: Behavioral Publications.

Carroll, J. (2000, January 2). And the sea is never full. *New York Times,* p. 10.

Chambers, C. A. (1986). Women in the creation of the profession of social work. *Social Service Review, 60*(2), 1–33.

Chau, K. L. (1991). *Ethnicity and biculturalism: Emerging perspectives in group work.* New York: Hayworth.

Clandinin, D. J., & Connelly, M. (2000). *Narrative inquiry.* San Francisco: Jossey-Bass.

Cohen, B. J. (1999). Fostering innovation in a large human service bureaucracy. *Administration in Social Work, 23*(2), 47–59.

Cohen, N. E. (1958). *Social work in the American tradition.* New York: Holt, Rinehart & Winston.

Coles, R. (1989). *The call of stories.* Boston: Houghton Mifflin.

Combs, G., & Freedman, J. (1998). Tellings and retellings. *Journal of Marital and Family Therapy, 24*(4), 405–413.

Connerton, P. (1989). *How societies remember.* New York: Cambridge University Press.

Coyle, G. (1962). Concepts relevant to helping the family as a group. *Social Casework, 41*(8), 347–355.

Coyle, G. L. (1958). *Social sciences in professional education.* New York: Council on Social Work Education.

De Anda, D. (1977). *Controversial issues in multiculturalism.* Boston: Allyn & Bacon.

de Shazer, S. (1982). *Patterns of brief family therapy.* New York: Norton.

Dean, R. G. (1998). A Narrative approach to groups. *Clinical Social Work Journal, 26*(1), 23–37.

Devine, E. T. (1922). *Social work.* New York: The Macmillan Company.

Devore, W., & Schlesinger, W. (1987). *Ethnic sensitive social work practice.* Columbus, OH: Merrill.

Dewey, J. (1957). *Reconstruction in philosophy.* Boston: Beacon.

Doan, R. (1998). The King is dead; Long live the king: Narrative therapy and practicing what we preach. *Family Process, 37*(3), 379–385.

Dyson, A. H. (1994). The ninjas, the x-men, and the ladies: Playing with power and identity in an urban primary school. *Teachers College Record, 96*(2), 22–30.

Eakin, E. (2000, January 15). Bigotry as mental illness or just another norm. *New York Times,* pp. 1, 31.

Eastland, L. S., Henderson, S., & Baron, J. (1999). *Communication in recovery.* Cresskill, NJ: Hampton Press.

Ellison, R. (1989). *Invisible man.* New York: Vintage.

Epston, D., & White, M. (1990). *Experience, contradiction, narrative & imagination: Selected papers.* South Australia: Dulwich Center Publications.

Epston, D., & Roth, S. (1994, Feb. 7). Framework for a White/Epston type interview. *Dulwich Center Publications,* 1–6.

Epston, D. (1996). Letter Writing Workshop. Los Angeles, CA.

Fanon, F. (1967). *Black skin, white masks.* New York: Grove.

Farley, M. (2000, February 10). Mental illness by mandate. *Los Angeles Times,* pp. 1, 20–21.

Flexner, A. (1915). Is social work a profession? *National Conference of Charities and Corrections.* Chicago: Hildman Printing Co.

Focht, L. (1996). "Speech after long silence": The use of narrative therapy in a preventive intervention for children of parents with affective disorders. *Family Process, 35,* 407–422.

Foucault, M. (1965). *Madness and civilization.* New York: Mentor Books.

Foucault, M. (1977). *Discipline and punish: The birth of the prison.* New York: Pantheon.

Foucault, M. (1978). *The history of sexuality, Vol 1.* New York: Pantheon.

Foucault, M. (1980). *Power/Knowledge: Selected interviews and other writings.* New York: Pantheon.

Freedman, J., & Combs, G. (1996). *Narrative therapy.* New York: Norton.

Friedman, J. (1973). *Retracking America.* New York: Anchor.

Friedman, S. E. (1993). *The new language of change: Constructive collaboration in psychotherapy.* New York: Guilford.

Gagerman, J. R. (1997). Integrating dream analysis with inter subjectivity in group psychotherapy. *Clinical Social Work Journal, 25*(2).

Gains, A. T. (1992). From DSM-1 to III-R; Voices of self mastery and the other: A cultural constructivist reading of U.S. psychiatric classification. *Social Science Medicine, 35*(1), 3–24.

Galinsky, M. J., & Schopler, J. H. (1995). *Support groups.* New York: Hayworth.

Garbarino, G. K., Kosteiny, K., & Dubroy, N. (1991). What children can tell us about living in danger. *American Psychologist, 46*(4), 376–383.

Gergan, K. T. (1985), The social constructivist movement in modern psychology. *American Psychologist, 40*(3), 255–275.

Germain, C. B. (1981). The ecological approach to people-environment transactions. *Social Casework, 62,* 323–331.

Germain, C. B., & Gitterman, A. (1980). *The life model of social work practice.* New York: Columbia University Press.

Gilligan, C. (1982). *In a different voice.* Cambridge, MA: Harvard University Press.

Gilligan, S., & Price, R. (Eds.). (1993). *Therapeutic conversations.* New York: Norton.

Gitterman, A., & Shulman, S. (1994). *Mutual aid groups, vulnerable populations and the life cycle.* New York: Columbia University Press.

Goffman, E. (1963). *Stigma.* Englewood Cliffs, NJ: Prentice Hall.

Goldstein, H. (1998). Different Families. *Families in Society, 802,* 107–109.

Goleman, D. (1998). *Working with emotional intelligence.* New York: Bantam.

Gordon, L. R. (1996). *Fanon: A critical reader.* Malden, MA: Blackwell.

Gorman, J. (1993). Postmodernism and the conduct of inquiry in social work. *Affilia, 8*(3), 247–265.

Gottlieb, A. (1997, January). Crisis of consciousness. *Unte Reader, 45–48.*

Green, J. (1982). *Cultural awareness in the human services.* Englewood Cliffs, NJ: Prentice Hall.

Green, J. W. (1995). *Cultural awareness in the human services* (2nd ed.). Boston: Allyn & Bacon.

Guernsey, L. (1999, Dec. 16). The web: New ticket to a pink slip. *New York Times,* pp. 1, 8.

Haley, J. (1971). *The power tactics of Jesus Christ.* New York: Avon.

Haley, S. A. (1974). When the patient reports atrocities. *Archives of General Psychiatry, 30,* 191–196.

Hamlet, J. D. (1994). Religious discourse as cultural narrative: A critical analysis of African-American sermons. *The Western Journal of Black Studies, 18*(1), 11–17.

Hart, B. (1995). Re-authoring the stories we work by. *Australian and New Zealand Journal of Family Therapy, 16*(4), 181–189.

Hartman, A., & Laird, J. (1983). *Family centered social work practice.* New York: Free Press.

Heineman, M. (1981). The obsolete scientific imperative in social work research and practice. *Social Service Review, 56*(3), 371–396.

Hoffman, L. (1998). Setting aside the model in family therapy. *Journal of Marital and Family Therapy, 24*(2), 145–156.

Holland, T. (1991). Narrative knowledge and professional practice. *Social Thought, 17*(1).

Holland, T. P., & Kilpatrick, A. C. (1993). Using narrative techniques to enhance multicultural practice. *Journal of Social Work Education, 29*(3), 302–309.

Holmes, T. H., & Rahe, H. (1967). The Social readjustment scale. *Journal of Psychosomatic Research, 11,* 213.

Hoyt, M. (Ed.). (1966). *Constructive therapies 2.* New York: Guilford.

Illich, I. (1973). *Tools for conviviality.* New York: Harper & Row.

Illich, I. (1975). *Medical nemeses.* Mexico: CIDOC.

Johnson, A. G. (1995). *The Blackwell dictionary of sociology.* Malden, MA: Blackwell.

Kagle, J. D. (1987). Recording in direct practice. *Encyclopedia of social work* (18 ed., Vol. II., pp. 463–467). Silver Spring, MD: NASW.

Karenga, M. (1998). *Kwanza.* Los Angeles: University of Sankore.

Katz, A. H. (1970). Self-help organizations and volunteer participation in social work. *Social Work, 18*(3), 51–60.

Katz, A. H. (1993). *Self-help in America.* New York: Twayn Publishers.

Kellman, S. G. (1985). *Approaches to teaching Camus' The plague.* New York: Modern Language Association of America.

Kilpatrick, A., & Holland, T. P. (1995). *Working with families.* Boston: Allyn & Bacon.

Kozol, J. (1995). *Amazing Grace.* New York: Harper.

Krog, A. (1998). *Country of my skull.* Random House: Johannesburg, South Africa.

Kropotkin, P. A. (1972). *Mutual aid a foundation of evolution.* New York: New York University Press.

Kuczynski, A. (2000, January 6). Radio squeezes empty air space for profit. *New York Times,* p. 1.

Laird, J. (1995). Family-centered practice in the postmodern era. *Families in Society, 76*(3), 150–162.

Laird, J. (1993). *Revisioning social work education: A social constructionist approach.* New York: Hayworth.

Langellier, K. M., & Peterson, J. (1994). Family story telling as a strategy of social control. In D. K. Mumby (Ed.), *Narrative and social control: Critical perspectives.* Newbury Park, CA: Sage.

Laube, J. J., & Trefz, H. (1994). Group therapy using a narrative theory framework. *Journal of Systemic Therapies, 13*(2), 29–37.

Lawson, D. M, & Prevatt, F. (1999). *Casebook in family therapy.* Belmont, CA: Brooks Cole.

Lee, J. A. B. (1994). *The empowerment approach to social work practice.* New York: Columbia University Press.

Lefkowitz, M. (1996). *Not out of Africa.* New York: Basic.

LeShan, L. (1997). The DSM21: Introduction. *Advances: The Journal of Mind-Body Health, 13*(3), 67.

Levine, J. E. (1997). Re-Visioning attention deficit hyperactivity disorder (ADHD). *Clinical Social Work Journal, 25*(2), 197–209.

Lewin, K. (1958). *Group decision and social change.* New York: Holt.

Liebow, E. (1993). *Tell them who I am: The lives of homeless women.* New York: Free Press.

Link, R. J., & Sullivan, M. (1988). Vital connections: Using literature to illustrate social work issues. *Social Work Education, 25*(3), 192–230.

Lippitt, R., Watson, J., & Westly, B. (1958). *The dynamics of planned change.* New York: Harcourt Brace.

Llosa, M. V. (1989). *The story teller.* New York: Penguin.

Lorber, J., & Satow, R. (1977). Creating a company of unequals. *Sociology of Work and Occupations, 4*(3), 281–301.

Lubove, R. (1965). *The professional altruist.* Cambridge, MA: Harvard University Press.

Ludy, T. J., & Diyon, D. N. (1996). Dream analysis by mail: An American woman seeks Freud's advice. *American Psychologist, 51*(5), 461–468.

Lysack, M. (1995). Narrative therapy with incarcerated teenagers and their families. *The Family Side of Corrections, 7*(2), 1–4.

Madigan, S. (1993). Questions about questions. In S. Gilligan (Ed.), *Therapeutic Conversations.* New York: Norton.

Madigan, S. (1996). The politics of identity. *Journal of Systemic Therapies, 15*(1), 47–62.

Marin, P. (1981, Nov.). Living in moral pain. *Psychology Today, (13)*1, 68–80.

Martin, J. C. (1992). Therapists' intentional use of metaphor: Memorability, clinical impact, and possible epistemic/motivational functions. *Journal of Consulting and Clinical Psychology, 60,* 143–145.

McKinlay, A., & Starkey, K. (1997). *Foucault, management and organization theory.* London: Sage.

McNamee, S., & Gergan, K. (1992). *Therapy as social construction.* Thousand Oaks, CA: Sage.

McQuade, S. (1999). Using psychodynamic, cognitive-behavioral and solution-focused questioning to co-construct a new narrative. *Clinical Social Work Journal, 27*(4), 339–353.

Meyer, C. (1976). *Social work practice.* New York: Free Press.

Michell, J. F. (1983). *The new view over Atlantis.* San Francisco: Harper.

Miller, J. (1995). A narrative interview with Mitchell Ginsberg. *Reflections: Narratives of Professional Helping, 1*(3), 44–63.

Miller, J. (1999). A narrative interview with Ann Hartman: Part three: Keeping the social in social work. *Reflections: Narratives of Professional Helping, 5*(1), 60–70.

Mills, C. W. (1959). *The sociological imagination.* New York: Oxford University Press.

Minuchin, S. (1974). *Families and family therapy.* Cambridge, MA: Harvard University Press.

Minuchin, S. (1991). The seduction of constructionism. *Family Networker, 15*(5), 47–50.

Minuchin, S. (1998). Where is the family in narrative family therapy? *Journal of Marital and Family Therapy, 24*(4), 397–403.

Minuchin, S. (1999). Retelling, re-imagining, and re-searching: A continuing conversation. *Journal of Marital and Family Therapy, 25*(1), 9–14.

Monk, G., Winside, J., Crocket, K., & Epston, D. (1997). *Narrative Therapy in practice: The archaeology of hope.* San Francisco: Jossey-Bass.

Moreno, J. L. (1934). *Who shall survive?* Washington, DC: Nervous and Mental Disease Publishing Co.

Morgan, A. (2000). *What is narrative therapy?* Adelade, South Australia: Dulwich Centre Publications.

Mumby, D. K. (1994). *Narrative therapy and social control: Critical perspectives.* Newbury Park, CA: Sage

Myerhoff, B. (1982). Life history among the elderly: Performance, visibility and remembering. In J. Ruby (Ed.), *A crack in the mirror*. Philadelphia: University of Pennsylvania Press.

Myrdal, G. (1962). *An American dilemma*. New York: Harper & Row.

Nichols, M. P., & Schwartz, R. C. (1998). *Family Therapy* (4th ed.). Boston: Allyn & Bacon.

Niebuhr, G. (1999, Sept. 5). Priest rebuked by Vatican resumes public speaking. *New York Times*, p. 19.

Norton, A. (Ed.). (1994). *Dictionary of ideas*. London: Brockhampton Press.

Nylund, D. (1994). The economics of narrative. *The Family Therapy Networker, 18*(6), 39–39.

O'Hanlon, B. (1994). The third wave. *The Family Therapy Networker, 18*(6), 19–29.

O'Hara, M. (1995). Constructing emancipating realities. In W. T. Anderson (Ed.), *The truth about truth: De-confusing and re-constructing the post-modern world*. New York: G. P. Putnam.

Okin, S. M. (1999). *Is multiculturalism bad for women?* Princeton, NJ: Princeton University Press.

Onesto, L. (1997). In memory, Toni Cade Bambara: Passing on the story. *The Black Scholar, 26*(2), 42–46.

Papell, C., & Rothman, B. (1966). Social group work models: Possession and heritage. *Journal of Education for Social Work, 2*, 66–77.

Parry, A., & Doan, R. B. (1994). *Story revisions: narrative therapy in the postmodern world*. New York: Guilford.

Pear, R. (2000, April 30). Research neglects women, studies find. *New York Times*, p. 20.

Perlman, H. (1957). *Social casework: A problem solving process*. Chicago: University of Chicago Press.

Piercy, M. (1980). *The moon is always female*. New York: Knopf.

Pinderhughes, E. (1995). Empowering diverse populations: Family practice in the 21st century. *Families in Society: The Journal of Contemporary Human Services, 76*(3), 131–140.

Piven, F. F., & Cloward, R. A. (1971). *Regulating the poor: The functions of public welfare*. New York: Vintage.

Polkinghorne, D. (1988). *Narrative knowing and the human sciences*. New York: Albany State Press.

Progoff, I. (1975). *At a journal workshop: The basic guide for using the intensive journal*. New York: Dialogue House Library.

Pumphrey, R. E., & Pumphrey, M. W. (1956). *The heritage of American social work*. New York: Columbia University Press.

Putnam, R. D. (2000). *Bowling Alone*. New York: Simon & Shuster.

Quinones, E. (1999, Aug. 1). *New York Times*, Sec 3, p. 4.

Rambo, A. H. (1993). *Practicing therapy*. New York: Guilford.

Rasheed, J. M., & Rasheed, M. (1999). *Social Work practice with African American men*. Thousand Oaks, CA: Sage.

Reynolds, B. C. (1931). A way of understanding. *The Family, 12*(7), 203–292.

Reynolds, B. (1934). *Between client and community.* New York: Oriole Editions.

Reynolds, B. (1965). *Learning and teaching in the practice of Social Work.* New York: Russell & Russell.

Rhodes, C. (1997). The legitimation of learning in organizational change. *Journal of Organizational Change Management, 10*(1), 10–20.

Rhodes, W. A., & Brown, W. K. (1991). *Why some children succeed despite the odds.* New York: Praeger.

Richmond, M. (1917). *Social diagnosis.* New York: Russell Sage Foundation.

Riesman, F. (1976). How does self help work? *Social Policy, 7*, 41–45.

Robinson, V. (1930). *A changing psychology in social case work.* Chapel Hill, NC: University of North Carolina Press.

Romme, A. J. (1989). Hearing voices. *Schizophrenia Bulletin, 15*, 209–216.

Rosenzweig, R., & Thelen, T. (1998). *The presence of the past.* New York Columbia University Press.

Ruby, J. E. (1982). *A crack in the mirror.* Philadelphia: University of Pennsylvania Press.

Saleebey, D. (1992). *The strength perspective in social work practice.* New York: Longman.

Saleebey, D. (1994). Culture, theory and narrative: The intersection of meaning and practice. *Social Work, 39*(4), 351–359.

Sampson, T. (1999). The welfare rights movement. *Social Policy, 30*(2), 51–53.

Schon, D. A. (1983). *The reflective practitioner.* New York: Basic.

Schwartz, R. C. (1999). Narrative therapy expands and contracts family therapy's horizons. *Journal of Marital and Family Therapy, 25*(2), 263–267.

Schwartz, W. (1961). The social worker in the group. *Proceedings National Conference on Social Welfare.* New York: Columbia University Press.

Schwartz, W. (1974). Private troubles and public issues: One social work or two? In P. Weinberger (Ed.), *Perspectives on social welfare* (2nd ed.). New York: MacMillan.

Shah, I. (1981). *Learning to learn psychology and spirituality the Sufi way.* Cambridge: Harper & Row.

Shatan, C. F. (1973). The grief of soldiers. *American Journal of Orthopsychiatry, 43*(4), 640–653.

Sharkey, J. (1997, Sept. 28). You're not bad, you're sick: It's in the book. *New York Times*, pp. 1, 5.

Sherif, M. (1969). *Social Psychology.* New York: Harper & Row.

Shulman, L. (1992). *The skills of helping: Individuals families and groups.* Itaska, IL: Peacock.

Sluzki, C. E. (1998). In search of the lost family: A footnote to Minuchin's essay. *Journal of Marital and Family Therapy, 24*(4), 415–417.

Specht, H., & Courtney, M. E. (1993). *Unfaithful angels: How social work abandoned its mission.* New York: Free Press.

Spence, D. P. (1984). *Narrative truth and historical truth: Meaning and interpretation in psychoanalysis*. New York: Norton.

Spence, D. P. (1987). *The Freudian metaphor*. New York: Norton.

Spolin, V. (1963). *Improvisation for the theater*. Evanston, IL: Northwestern University Press.

Stacey, K. (1994). Language as an exclusive or inclusive concept: Reaching beyond the verbal. *Annals of the New Zealand Journal of Family Therapy, 16*(3), 123–132.

Stacey, K., & Loptson, C. (1995). Children should be seen and not heard? *Journal of Systemic Therapies, 14*(4), 16–31.

Stark, E. (1979). Medicine and patriarchal violence. *International Journal of Health Service, 9*(3), 461–493.

Stern, S. D., & Szmukler, G. L. (1999). Disruption and reconstruction: Narrative insights into the experience of family members caring for a relative with serious mental illness. *Family Process, 38*(1), 353–369.

Taft, J. (1933). *The dynamics of therapy in a controlled relationship*. New York: MacMillan.

Talbot, M. (2000, Jan. 9). The placebo connections. *New York Times*, Magazine, pp. 12–17.

Tamaki, J. (1998, July 13). Cultural balancing act adds to teen angst. *Los Angeles Times*, pp. 1, 10, 11.

Tandy, C., & Gallant, J. P. (1993). *Narrative therapy a case study*. Unpublished manuscript, The University of Georgia School of Social Work. Athens, Georgia.

Taylor, F. (1911). *Scientific management*. New York: Harper & Row.

Tomm, K. (1998). A question of perspective. *Journal of Marital and Family Therapy, 24*(4), 409–413.

Turkewitz, G., & Dorenny, D. A. (1993). *Developmental time and timing*. Hillsdale, NJ: Lawrence Erlbaum.

Tweed Valley Health Service. (1996). *Narrative therapy in action*. Agency Announcement. New Zealand.

van Dijk, T. A. Stories and racism. In D. K. Mumby (Ed.), *Narrative and social control: Critical perspectives*. Newbury Park, CA: Sage.

Wakefield, J. C. (1996). Does social work need the ecosystems perspective? *Social Service Review, 70*(2), 1–31.

Walkowitz, D. J. (1999). *Working with class: Social workers and the politics of middle-class identity*. Chapel Hill, NC: University of North Carolina Press.

Warner, A. G. (1889). Scientific charity. *The Popular Science Monthly, 35*, 488–493.

Warner, A. J. (1894). *American characteristics and social work*. New York: Macmillan.

Weaver, H. N. (1999). Indigenous people and the social work profession: Defining culturally competent services. *Social Work, 44*(3), 217–225.

Weick, A. (1993). Reconstructing social work education. In J. Laird (Ed.), *Revisioning social work education.* New York: Haworth.

Weick, K. E. (1993). The collapse of sensemaking in organizations: The Mann Gulch disaster. *Administrative Science Quarterly, 31,* 628–652.

Weingarten, K. (2000). Witnessing, wonder and hope. *Family Process, 39*(4), 389–402.

Weiss, T. G., & Minear, L. (1993). *Humanitarianism across borders.* Boulder, CO: Lynne Riener.

Wheelis, A. (1973). *How people change.* New York: Harper.

White, C. (1995). Speaking out and being heard. *Dulwich Center Newsletter, 4,* 1–54.

White, M. (1989, Spring). The externalization of the problem and the re-authoring of lives and relationships. *Dulwich Center Newsletter,* 7–11.

White, M. (1989). *Selected papers.* Adelaide, Australia: Dulwich Center Publications.

White, M. (1991). Deconstruction and therapy. *Dulwich Centre Newsletter, 3,* 1–21.

White, M. (1994). *The politics of therapy.* Adelaide, South Australia: Dulwich Center Publications.

White, M. (1995a). *Re-Authoring lives: interviews and essays.* Adelaide, South Australia: Dulwich Center Publications.

White, M. (1995b). Externalizing conversation exercise. *Dulwich Center Newsletter,* October, 1–3

White, M., & Epston, D. (1990). *Narrative means to therapeutic ends.* New York: Norton.

Whittaker, J. K., & Garbarino, J. (1983). *Social support networks.* New York: Aldine.

Wines, M. (2000, December 31). A fit city offers Russia a self-help model. *New York Times,* pp. 1, 10.

Woodroofe, K. (1962). *From charity to social work: In England and the United States.* London: Routledge and Kegan Paul.

Woods, R. A. (1894). University settlements: Laboratories in social science. *Proceedings, International Congress of Charities, Corrections, and Philanthropy. Chicago, June 1993* (pp. 23–24). Baltimore: John Hopkins University Press.

Woods, R. A. (1905). Social work a new profession. *International Journal of Ethics, XVI,* 25–39.

Woods, R. A. (1970). *The neighborhood in nation-building.* New York: Arno Press.

Wuthnow, R. (1998). *Loose connections.* Cambridge, MA: Harvard University Press.

Yalom, I. D. (1980). *Existential psychotherapy.* New York: Basic.

Yalom, I. D. (1995). *The theory and practice of group psychotherapy.* New York: Basic.

Yalom, I. D. (1998). *The Yalom reader.* New York: Basic.

Zimmerman, T. S., & Sheperd, R. (1993). Externalizing the problem of Bulimia: Conversation, drawing and letter writing in group therapy. *Journal of Systemic Therapies, 12*(1), 22–31.

Zimmerman, J. L., & Dickerson, V. C. (1993). Using a narrative metaphor: Implications for theory and clinical practice. *Family Process, 33,* 235–245.

Index